The Manual of
Trigger Point *and*
Myofascial Therapy

The Manual of
Trigger Point *and*
Myofascial Therapy

Dimitrios Kostopoulos, PT, PhD

Konstantine Rizopoulos, PT, FABS

Hands-On Physical Therapy, PC
Astoria, New York

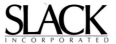

SLACK
INCORPORATED

an innovative information, education, and management company
6900 Grove Road • Thorofare, NJ 08086

Publisher: John H. Bond
Editorial Director: Amy E. Drummond
Senior Associate Editor: Jennifer Stewart
Part B photographs by: Kosmas Kokkaris
Referred pain pattern illustrations by: Bonnie Mousis
Anatomical illustrations by: Hands-On Physical Therapy and adapted by Nick Fasnacht

The procedures and practices described in this book should be implemented in a manner consistent with the professional standards set for the circumstances that apply in each specific situation. Every effort has been made to confirm the accuracy of the information presented and to correctly relate generally accepted practices. The author, editor, and publisher cannot accept responsibility for errors or exclusions or for the outcome of the application of the material presented herein. There is no expressed or implied warranty of this book or information imparted by it. Any review or mention of specific companies or products is not intended as an endorsement by the author or the publisher.

The work SLACK publishes is peer reviewed. Prior to publication, recognized leaders in the field, educators, and clinicians provide important feedback on the concepts and content that we publish. We welcome feedback on this work.

Kostopoulos, Dimitrios.
    The manual of trigger point and myofascial therapy / Dimitrios Kostopoulos, Konstantine Rizopoulos ; foreword, Reuben S. Ingber.
        p. ; cm.
    Includes bibliographical references and index.
    ISBN 1-55642-542-2 (alk. paper)
    Hard cover ISBN 1-55642-549-X
    1. Myofascial pain syndromes--Physical therapy. I. Title: Manual of trigger point and myofascial therapy.
II. Rizopoulos, Konstantine. III. Title.
    [DNLM: 1. Myofascial Pain Syndromes--therapy. 2. Physical Therapy. WE 550 K86m 2001]
RC927.3 .K67 2001
616.7'4--dc21
                                                                                    2001031122

Printed in the United States of America

Published by: SLACK Incorporated
                   6900 Grove Road
                   Thorofare, NJ 08086 USA
                   Telephone: 856-848-1000
                   Fax: 856-853-5991
                   www.slackbooks.com

    Contact SLACK Incorporated for more information about other books in this field or about the availability of our books from distributors outside the United States.
    Authorization to photocopy items for internal or personal use, or the internal or personal use of specific clients, is granted by SLACK Incorporated, provided that the appropriate fee is paid directly to Copyright Clearance Center, 222 Rosewood Drive, Danvers, MA 01923 USA, 978-750-8400. Prior to photocopying items for educational classroom use, please contact the CCC at the address above. Please reference Account Number 9106324 for SLACK Incorporated's Professional Book Division.
    For further information on CCC, check CCC Online at the following address: http://www.copyright.com.

    Last digit is print number: 10 9 8 7 6 5 4 3 2 1

CONTENTS

Shoulder Region

Upper Extremity Region

Abdominal Region

Thoracolumbar Spine Region

Lumbar Spine Region

Lower Extremity Region

Adductor Magnus 190
Pectineus 192
Tensor Fasciae Latae 194
Rectus Femoris 196
Vastus Medialis 198
Vastus Lateralis 200
Vastus Intermedius 202
Biceps Femoris (Long and Short Heads) 204
Semitendinosus and Semimembranosus 206
Popliteus 208
Gastrocnemius 210
Soleus 212
Tibialis Anterior 214
Tibialis Posterior 216
Peroneus Longus 218
Peroneus Brevis 220
Peroneus Tertius 222
Extensor Digitorum Brevis 224
Flexor Hallucis Brevis 226
Flexor Digitorum Brevis 228
Quadratus Plantae 230
Adductor Hallucis 232

Index 235

Acknowledgments

It seems that the Acknowledgments is the toughest section of the book to write considering the reality that some people will inevitably be left out.

We would like to start by thanking all those who have contributed and still contribute to helping us find our professional and personal paths in life.

We are grateful to our parents Eleni and Constantine Kostopoulos and Despina and Dimitrios Rizopoulos, to whom we owe everything we are today. Bonnie and Tom, thank you for the ongoing support especially during those stressful moments. Special thanks to George Mousis for his modeling, which appears in the photographs throughout the book. Christine Salmon and Wessel Oosthuizen, thanks for your encouragement and help, especially when covering us by treating patients when we had publisher's deadlines to meet.

We are thankful to several people who have shaped our professional lives (order is irrelevant): Professors Apostolos Dumas and Panagiotis Giokaris; Drs. Reuben Ingber, Arthur Nelson, Claudette Lefebvre, Karel Lewit, Vladimir Janda, Rick Nielsen, John Upledger; and many others who have been our teachers and mentors.

We would like to acknowledge the memory of Dr. Doris Berryman, who will always be with us.

We would like to extend sincere respect and appreciation to the following people who have contributed to the area of myofascial dysfunction most of whom we have never met, yet we feel we have known them for years: Drs. Janet Travell, David Simons, Robert Gerwin, Mary Maloney, Robert Bennett, Chan Gunn, C. Hong, James Fricton, and many others.

Special thanks to John Bond, Amy Drummond, Jennifer Stewart, Carrie Kotlar, and the rest of the associates at SLACK Incorporated, as well as Nick Fasnacht at Kingfish Studios, who believed in our work and worked hard to meet deadlines.

It was a great pleasure for us to be involved in the writing of this book. We are proud to be physical therapists and to have the opportunity to share our skills, opinions, clinical experience, and expertise with our patients and colleagues. We have dedicated our professional lives to further research, exploration, education, and practice of manual therapy, especially myofascial therapy. We would like to thank our colleagues, students, friends, and coworkers, but most of all our patients, for their great tolerance, support, and encouragement in this exciting journey.

ABOUT THE AUTHORS

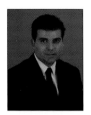 Dimitrios Kostopoulos, PT, PhD is the cofounder of Hands-On Physical Therapy. He earned his doctorate and master's degrees at New York University and is actively pursuing his second doctorate of science degree in clinical electrophysiology at Rocky Mountain University, Provo, Utah. Dr. Kostopoulos has extensive training and teaching experience in different areas of manual therapy, with emphasis in trigger point, myofascial, and neurofascial therapy, as well as manipulation. He is a past faculty member at Mercy College, Dobbs Ferry, NY, a diplomate of the American Academy of Pain Management, and an active member of the American Physical Therapy Association (APTA).

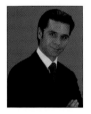 Konstantine Rizopoulos, PT, FABS is the cofounder of Hands-On Physical Therapy. He earned his undergraduate degree from the University of Athens, Greece and has completed extensive postgraduate studies in manual therapy. Mr. Rizopoulos has extensive experience in the area of manual therapy, particularly in myofascial and trigger point therapies and their application to neurologic and pediatric populations. He is an active member of the APTA, a fellow member of the American Back Society, and a member of the Hellenic Medical Society.

Dimitrios Kostopoulos and Konstantine Rizopoulos are the developers of a comprehensive therapeutic approach that integrates trigger point, myofascial, neurofascial, and proprioceptive therapy techniques, and they teach continuing education courses in the United States and Europe.

For more information on the authors' continuing education programs or for any other information, you may contact them at:

Hands-On Physical Therapy, PC
32-70 31st Street
Astoria, NY 11106
1-888-767-5003
(718) 626-2699
www.hands-on-pt.com

PREFACE

One of the most fascinating things in physical therapy, as well as other health professions—especially when dealing with pain—is to replace the agonizing, frustrating feeling of pain from the patients' faces with a feeling of comfort, relaxation, and hope.

* Pain is a fear experienced by all living creatures who are equipped with pain receptors
* Pain is counter to survival
* Pain is the number-one reason why a patient visits his or her doctor
* Pain has the power to affect all four major domains in people's lives: physical, emotional, mental, and social

ACCURATE DIAGNOSIS

The survival instinct is something all living organisms have in common; because pain is counter to survival, people try to create different mechanisms and strategies to avoid or alleviate pain. Others who feel hopeless and tired of fighting learn to live with pain.

Several health care professions deal with the diagnosis and treatment of pain and musculoskeletal dysfunction. It is apparent that to effectively treat a pathological condition, accuracy in diagnosis is essential. Despite the advances of medicine, especially in the area of "high-tech" diagnostic tools, accurate diagnosis sometimes becomes a big challenge for the clinician. A major cause of somatic, somatovisceral, and somatoemotional pain and dysfunction can be the myofascial trigger point syndrome. Although skeletal muscles account for 40% of the total body weight,[1] the musculoskeletal system is among the least studied in many medical schools. This may account for the large number of misdiagnoses related to myofascial pain. Physical therapists and other health care professionals study the musculoskeletal system in great detail; however, issues related to the myofascial trigger point syndrome are hardly mentioned in most clinical curricula. In most cases, clinicians are exposed to the condition for the first time at some point in their clinical affiliations, especially when other diagnoses and treatments have failed to resolve a patient's problem.

ACCURATE TREATMENT

When an accurate myofascial diagnosis is established, the challenge shifts to appropriate and efficient treatment. In our various teachings and presentations on the subject, it has become a cliché for us to mention to students over and over again the example of a patient who sees two different clinicians who both profess expertise in the field of myofascial pain and dysfunction. One of them succeeds in resolving the patient's problem while the other one fails. An intervention for such a syndrome goes beyond the establishment of a proper diagnosis. Appropriate and accurate treatment must take place on a consistent basis. Method of treatment, hand placement, handling of the needle (when indicated), position of myofascial stretching, and degree of stretching are all very important components to a successful treatment. Treatment errors that seem small may have an amplified negative effect on the patient. Reuben Ingber mentions that "overstretching even by 1 to 2 mm may not achieve the desired result and may cause increased symptoms."[2] We just recently evaluated a 55-year-old female patient who underwent two lumbar fusions. At this point she suffers from severe lower back, groin, and anterior thigh pain. One of the physicians tending to her problem suggested that she receive injections of botulinum A toxin in several areas of her lower back (lumbar paraspinal muscles). While the procedure may indeed have very positive results for this patient, it is still considered a rather invasive or, at least, aggressive type of intervention. One must be absolutely certain that the correct muscle(s) has been chosen before applying any kind of treatment to a patient, especially an invasive one. After examining this patient, it became apparent to us from the referred pain pattern (RPP) as well as from the rest of the evaluation and biomechanical analysis of movement that she exhibited active myofascial trigger points in her iliopsoas muscle. A series of treatments to the iliopsoas muscle completely resolved the symptoms and resolved proper function in the lumbar spine and pelvic areas. Obviously, application of botulinum A injections to the lumbar paraspinal muscles may not have had as positive an effect as the treatment to the iliopsoas muscle. The point of this scenario is to demonstrate that the clinician must be precise with the diagnosis and treatment interventions before any action is taken.

RESEARCH

Tremendous strides have been made during the past few years in the search for answers to the challenges surrounding myofascial trigger point syndrome. Research in the areas of histopathology and electrophysiology has provided us with substantial evidence regarding the pathogenesis and pathophysiology of myofascial trigger points. Neural science has supplied some answers to the burning questions surrounding referred pain patterns. Clinical studies in the area of reliability provide clinicians with greater confidence regarding the accuracy of the work we do. Unfortunately, there are those who have harmed the area of myofascial treatment with their "voodoo" approach to therapy. Without any scientific evidence and with nonspecific treatment protocols, they present their treatments as a panacea to any problem. "Just trust" and "just believe" attitudes do not belong to us. Through this textbook we open a forum for discussion and scientific exploration in the myofascial area. This is an open call for everyone interested to participate.

Dimitrios Kostopoulos, PT, PhD
Konstantine Rizopoulos, PT, FABS

REFERENCES

1. Silverthorn D. *Human Physiology: An Integrated Approach.* Upper Saddle Ridge, NJ: Prentice Hall; 1998.
2. Ingber R. *Myofascial Pain in Lumbar Dysfunction.* Philadelphia, Pa: Hanley & Belfus Inc; 1999.

FOREWORD

Health practitioners involved in musculoskeletal medicine are constantly searching for new and advanced methods of observation and analysis to facilitate learning and teaching. Myofascial dysfunction, introduced by Drs. Travell and Simons less than two decades ago, represents one of the newer methods of assessment and treatment. The mechanism and location of muscle injury have not been completely elucidated.

The authors provide some valuable insights into the assessment and treatment of a patient with musculoskeletal dysfunction. The addition of the concept of "biomechanics of injury" into the diagnostic assessment will be of great value to the practitioner and may even be useful in directing future research in the field. Kostopoulos and Rizopoulos' conceptual systematic approach is also found in the treatment of the dysfunctional muscle. To borrow from a pharmaceutical concept, there is a narrow therapeutic zone when stretching a muscle with myofascial dysfunction. Advising the patient as to the possible side effects, by being aware of the "positive stretch sign," is both easy to explain to the patient and essential to a positive outcome.

This book represents a significant development in the understanding of myofascial pain. Congratulations to the authors on their achievement. This volume will greatly contribute to the ever-growing body of knowledge on myofascial pain and will be a valuable addition to Travell and Simons' *Trigger Point Manual.*

Reuben S. Ingber, MD
Diplomate of the American Board of Physical Medicine and Rehabilitation
Past Chairman of the Myofascial Pain Special Interest Group of the
American Academy of Physical Medicine and Rehabilitation
New York, NY

ABOUT THE BOOK

This manual has been written in a format to serve both as a teaching textbook for the diagnosis and treatment of the myofascial trigger point syndrome, and as a clinical reference for the clinician interested in treating patients with such pathology.

The book is divided into two sections: the first section (Part A) covers the theory, current research, and trends regarding myofascial trigger point syndrome. In this section we review basic muscle and nerve physiology, which are important aspects in building a case for myofascial pathology. The pathogenesis of myofascial dysfunction, clinical symptoms and physical findings, as well as diagnostic criteria are explored through the most current research available. Treatment methods and techniques are then covered in a comprehensive, step-by-step manner.

An instructor using this textbook as a teaching resource is expected to teach this part chapter-by-chapter. Review questions are provided at the end of each chapter, which can help students test their level of understanding and identify areas that need to be studied further. An answer key is provided at the end of Part A.

The clinician is also expected to review Part A regardless of his or her level of expertise in order to obtain a better understanding of the various treatment methods.

The second section of the book (Part B) is divided into body regions. Each region includes those muscles that tend to have a higher incidence of myofascial involvement. The muscles are listed alphabetically in the Table of Contents for easy access. Comprehensive information for each muscle can be retrieved within two pages of text, illustrations, and photographs. This format can help the clinician save time when treating patients. Each muscle section includes information regarding muscle attachments (referenced here as origins and insertions to represent both open and closed chain movements), location of trigger points, referred pain patterns, myofascial stretching exercises, positive stretch signs, biomechanics of injury, and clinical notes when applicable. The location of the trigger points and referred pain patterns are illustrated with photographs. Photos are also provided for the myofascial trigger point treatment, the myofascial stretching exercises, and for home exercise programs. Various anatomical references were used for the origin, insertion, and relevant anatomy of the muscles studied. Location of myofascial trigger points and referred pain patterns have been retrieved through the reviewed literature as well as through the authors' clinical experience.

Note: The clinician's body positions in the photographs in this book do not represent correct and efficient ergonomics, but rather represent appropriate positions for effective illustration of the demonstrated techniques.

With no further delay, welcome to the exciting world of trigger point and myofascial therapy!

Part A

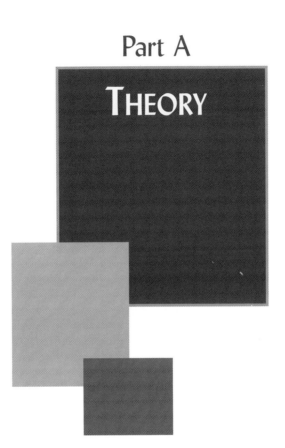

THEORY

Chapter 1

MYOFASCIAL TRIGGER POINTS: A HISTORICAL PERSPECTIVE

Looking back at the history and development of humankind, one may identify the genesis of myofascial trigger points in conjunction with the origins of our species. It seems that muscle microtrauma and presence of myofascial trigger points are consequences of our fight against gravity. Massaging a tender and painful spot within a muscle in order to provide relief is a common practice among people and has been known for thousands of years.

To gain a better understanding of the development of the myofascial trigger point syndrome, it is necessary to broaden our scope of defining terms and look at the similar meaning behind various kinds of terminology used to describe the same essentially pathological entity. Among the oldest known written texts that document sensitive skin areas and tender points on the human body are the texts of traditional Chinese medicine and acupuncture and later Japanese acupuncture texts.[1-3] Along the same lines are early recordings of manual medicine interventions dating back to the time of Hippocrates (400 BC).[4]

Froriep,[5] in the earlier part of the 19th century, identified tender, tight cords or bands within a muscle that produced pain. According to Lewit,[6] Gowers introduced the term *fibrositis* in 1904. Several other terms were introduced to describe the same type of phenomena, such as *myofibrositis, myalgia, myoangelosis, muscular rheumatism,* and others. In 1938, Kellgren[7] reported that various muscles in the body exhibit a characteristic referred pain pattern when injected with a salty solution. In the mid 1950s, Nimmo[8] introduced the soft tissue principles and trigger point interventions to the chiropractic profession. Nimmo was able to make the radical (for the chiropractic profession) conceptual leap from moving bones to working with muscles that move the bones.

The term *myofascial* did not appear in the medical literature until late 1940 when Travell, Gorell, Steindler, Rinzler,[9,10] and others started describing myofascial trigger areas in the lumbar spine to create *musculofascial pain*. In 1952, Dr. Travell[11] adopted the term *myofascial* after observing the referred pain pattern of the infraspinatus muscle during a muscle biopsy.

In 1983, Travell and Simons published the first volume of their trigger point manual entitled *Myofascial Pain and Dysfunction: The Trigger Point Manual*.[12] This was the first complete publication in the area of myofascial trigger point syndrome that identified specific trigger points, referred pain patterns, and perpetuating factors with a thorough review of the literature regarding the pathophysiology of trigger points. Travell and Simons, who are considered pioneers in the area of myofascial trigger point syndrome, published several other articles[13-18] establishing concise diagnostic and assessment criteria as well as treatment methods for myofascial dysfunction.

Around the same time, forerunners in rehabilitation medicine, Janda[19,20] and Lewit[6,21,22] from the Czech Republic, made significant contributions in establishing principles regarding muscle imbalances as well as alternate treatment methods for myofascial trigger points, such as the postisometric relaxation technique.[6,22]

During the early 1990s, Hubbard and others[23,24] reported various characteristics regarding the electromyographic activity of myofascial trigger points, while Simons and Hong[25-27] reached several conclusions regarding the pathophysiology of myofascial trigger points. Simons et al, in the recent publication of *The Trigger Point Manual*,[10] presented the most comprehensive review of the myofascial trigger point phenomena to date and established specific essential and confirmatory criteria for identifying

AUTHORS' CONTRIBUTION

The authors of this book have contributed to the field of myofascial trigger point syndrome through the development of various concepts within the past several years. These concepts include:

* **Biomechanics of Injury:**[29,30] A very important component in the diagnosis of trigger point myofascial syndrome, especially when a decision must be made regarding the appropriate muscle to treat. In other words, the specific mechanism that may be responsible for the injury must be considered. This includes direction of force, relative position of the body, and other parameters that will be further discussed in subsequent chapters.

* **Integration Model and Neurofascial Integration:** An evaluation and treatment model has been created that provides the ability to integrate the myofascial trigger point principles with the rest of the important systems of the body. Trigger points are not viewed as isolated entities within a muscle, but rather as dynamic pathological components that influence and are influenced by other components of the living organism, especially the central and peripheral nervous systems. The role of the nervous system in the development and continuous existence of myofascial trigger points is of great importance. At the same time, a myofascial trigger point may affect the nervous system either through biomechanical adaptations and compensatory mechanisms during locomotion or by direct mechanical effects in the neurofascia.

* **Positive Stretch Sign (PSS):**[30] A PSS is a pain indicator that allows the treating practitioner to identify the appropriate amount of myofascial stretch that should be applied to the muscle. The PSS concept was introduced by Ingber[31-34] and further established by the authors of this book for each of the muscles presented.

It is evident that future studies and publications will address myofascial trigger points both from a microcosmic as well as macrocosmic point of view. Future discoveries will confirm the origins and pathogenesis of the myofascial trigger point, while more objective and accurate methods for identification of trigger points will be developed. At the same time, there is a need for further exploration and integration of the myofascial trigger point syndrome with the central nervous system, its function, and pathology. This will lead to integrative, comprehensive treatments that will approach the body as a whole and not as a compartmentalized entity.

Bonica[35-38] suggested that acute pain has source peripheral structures that may be identifiable and treatable. On the other hand, *chronic pain syndrome*[39] is a result of dysfunction in the cortex,[35-38,40-43] especially the parietal lobe. Chronic pain syndrome may also include a peripheral component. The role of the clinician should be to prevent or delay the development of pain patterns in the brain cortex.[44,45] Once such pain patterns are fixed in the brain cortex, it becomes difficult or impossible to change them.

Trigger point and myofascial therapy will offer a possible solution for the management and/or resolution of such peripheral pain.

---

active and latent trigger points. Another very important step toward accurate identification of myofascial trigger points and their characteristics was a study by Gerwin et al.[28] They demonstrated a high degree of interrater reliability in identification of myofascial trigger point criteria.

REVIEW QUESTIONS

1. Gowers introduced the term *myofascial trigger point syndrome*.
   True   False

2. Travell and Simons introduced referred pain patterns and perpetuating factors for the various muscles.
   True   False

3. What technique did Lewit introduce for the treatment of myofascial trigger points?

REFERENCES

1. Ellis A, Wiseman N, Boss K. *Fundamentals of Chinese Acupuncture*. Brookline, Mass: Paradigm Publications; 1991.

2. O'Connor J, Bensky D. *Acupuncture: A Comprehensive Text. Shanghai College Of Traditional Medicine*. Seattle, Wash: Eastland Press, Inc; 1981.

3. Serizawa K. *Tsubo Vital Points for Oriental Therapy*. Tokyo: Japan Publications; 1976.

4. Schoitz EH. Manipulation treatment of the spinal column from the medical-historical standpoint. *Journal of the Norwegian Medical Association*. 1958;78:359-372.

5. Froriep R. *Ein Beitrag Zur Pathologie Und Therapie Des Rheumatismus*. Weimar, Germany: 1843.

6. Lewit K. *Manipulative Therapy in Rehabilitation of the Locomotor System*. Oxford, England: Butterworth-Heinemann; 1999.

7. Kellgren HJ. Observations on referred pain arising from muscle. *Clin Sci*. 1938;3:175-190.

8. Cohen JH, Gibbons RW. Raymond L. Nimmo and the evolution of trigger point therapy, 1929-1986. *J Manipulative Physiol Ther*. 1998;21:167-72.

9. Travell JG, Rinzler S, Herman M. Pain and disability of the shoulder and arm: treatment by intramuscular infiltration with procaine hydrochloride. *JAMA*. 1942;120:417-422.

10. Travell JG, Simons DG, Simons LS. *Myofascial Pain and Dysfunction: The Trigger Point Manual—Upper Half of Body*. Baltimore, Md: Williams & Wilkins; 1999.

11. Travell JG, Rinzler S. The myofascial genesis of pain. *Postgrad Med*. 1952;11:425-434.

12. Travell JG, Simons DG. *Myofascial Pain and Dysfunction: The Trigger Point Manual*. Vol 1. Baltimore, Md: Williams & Wilkins; 1983.

13. Simons DG. Myofascial pain syndromes. *Arch Phys Med Rehabil*. 1984;65:561.

14. Simons DG. Myofascial pain syndromes: where are we? where are we going? *Arch Phys Med Rehabil*. 1988;69:207-12.

15. Simons DG, Travell JG. Myofascial origins of low back pain. 1. Principles of diagnosis and treatment. *Postgrad Med*. 1983;73:66, 68-70.

16. Simons DG, Travell JG. Myofascial origins of low back pain. 2. Torso muscles. *Postgrad Med*. 1983;73:81-92.

17. Simons DG, Travell JG. Myofascial origins of low back pain. 3. Pelvic and lower extremity muscles. *Postgrad Med*. 1983;73:99-105, 108.

18. Travell JG, Simons DG. *Myofascial Pain and Dysfunction: The Trigger Point Manual—The Lower Extremities*. Media, Pa: Williams & Wilkins; 1983.

19. Janda V. Muscle strength in relation to muscle length, pain and muscle imbalance. *International Perspectives in Physical Therapy*. New York: Churchill Livingstone; 1993;8:83-91.

20. Twomey L, Janda V. *Physical Therapy of the Low Back: Muscles and Motor Control in Low Back Pain: Assessment and Management*. New York: Churchill Livingstone; 253-278.

21. Lewit K. The needle effect in the relief of myofascial pain. *Pain*. 1979;6:83-90.

22. Lewit K, Simons DG. Myofascial pain: relief by post-isometric relaxation. *Arch Phys Med Rehabil*. 1984;65:452-6.

23. Hubbard DR, Berkoff GM. Myofascial trigger points show spontaneous needle EMG activity. *Spine*. 1993;18:1803-7.

24. McNulty WH, Gevirtz RN, Hubbard DR, Berkoff GM. Needle electromyographic evaluation of trigger point response to a psychological stressor. *Psychophysiology*. 1994;31:313-6.

25. Hong CZ. Pathophysiology of myofascial trigger point. *J Formos Med Assoc*. 1996;95:93-104.

26. Hong CZ, Kuan TS, Chen JT, Chen SM. Referred pain elicited by palpation and by needling of myofascial trigger points: a comparison. *Arch Phys Med Rehabil*. 1997;78:957-60.

27. Hong CZ, Simons DG. Pathophysiologic and electrophysiologic mechanisms of myofascial trigger points. *Arch Phys Med Rehabil*. 1998;79:863-72.

28. Gerwin R, Shannon S. Interexaminer reliability and myofascial trigger points. *Arch Phys Med Rehabil*. 2000;81:1257-8.

29. Kostopoulos D, Rizopoulos K. Trigger point and myofascial therapy. *Advance for Physical Therapists*. 1998;6(15):25-28.

30. Kostopoulos D, Rizopoulos K, Brown A. Shin splint pain: the runner's nemesis. *Advance for Physical Therapists*. 1999;10(11):33-34.

31. Ingber RS. Iliopsoas myofascial dysfunction: a treatable cause of "failed" low back syndrome. *Arch Phys Med Rehabil*. 1989;70:382-6.

32. Ingber RS. Shoulder impingement in tennis/racquetball players treated with subscapularis myofascial treatments. *Arch Phys Med Rehabil*. 2000;81:679-82.

33. Ingber R. Personal communication; 1991.

34. Ingber R. *Myofascial Pain in Lumbar Dysfunction*. Philadelphia, Pa: Hanley & Belfus Inc; 1999.

35. Bonica JJ. Current concepts of the pain process. *Northwest Med*. 1970;69:661-4.

36. Bonica JJ. Neurophysiologic and pathologic aspects of acute and chronic pain. *Arch Surg*. 1977;112:750-61.

37. Bonica JJ. Pain: introduction. *Res Publ Assoc Res Nerv Ment Dis*. 1980;58:1-17.

38. Bonica JJ. Pain. *Triangle*. 1981;20:1-6.

39. Pilowsky I, Chapman CR, Bonica JJ. Pain, depression, and illness behavior in a pain clinic population. *Pain*. 1977;4:183-92.

40. Bonica JJ. Pain—basic principles of management. *Northwest Med*. 1970;69:567-8.

41. Bonica JJ. Neurophysiological and structural aspects of acute and chronic pain. *Recenti Prog Med*. 1976;61:450-75.

42. Bonica JJ. Basic principles in managing chronic pain. *Arch Surg*. 1977;112:783-8.

43. Bonica JJ. History of pain concepts and pain therapy. *Mt Sinai J Med*. 1991;58:191-202.

44. Janda V. Personal communication; 2000.

45. Janda V, Va'Vrota M. Sensory motor stimulation. In: Liebenson C. *Rehabilitation of the Spine*. Baltimore, Md: Williams & Wilkins; 1996:319-328.

Chapter 2

ACUPUNCTURE VERSUS TRIGGER POINT THERAPY

Clarification of the distinct differences between acupuncture and trigger point therapy is essential and useful both for health care professionals and for the public. Unfortunately, a number of acupuncture practitioners use a modified version in their definition of acupuncture points, which could be also defined as trigger points. This creates confusion in terms of appropriateness of treatment, which may have negative consequences when consumers have to make a decision as to who is the appropriate health care provider to treat their condition and what is the appropriate treatment for their condition. Belgrade[1-3] supports that "tender points are acupuncture points and can be often chosen for therapy." In other words, Belgrade uses one of the major criteria utilized to define a trigger point to also define an acupuncture point. Issues become even more confusing when one considers that trigger point dry needling,[4-6] one of the major treatments for myofascial trigger points, is performed with the use of an acupuncture needle. It is therefore imperative that a clear distinction is made between acupuncture and myofascial trigger points.

Acupuncture is a traditional system of Chinese medicine that has been practiced for more than 2000 years.[7] In some manner, the ancient Chinese became aware of certain sensitive skin areas (sensitive points) when a body organ, muscle, or function was impaired. They also observed that these sensitive skin areas were the same or similar in all people who suffered from the same impairment. Moreover, the sensitive areas varied consistently according to the organ or muscle function deviating from the norm. It was at this point that some of the relationships among various internal organs or muscles and their functions were observed and established.[7-9]

Acupuncture was introduced to the West in the 17th century by Jesuit missionaries sent to Peking. In the 1940s, the French sinologist and diplomat Soulie de Morant published his voluminous writings on acupuncture.[8] Acupuncture was first introduced in the United States in the late 1960s. Since then, Western licensed acupuncturists use acupuncture primarily for the relief of pain and other medical conditions. Melzack et al[10] found a 71% correlation between trigger points and acupuncture points for the treatment of pain. Melzack's contention was that trigger points and acupuncture points may have the same neural mechanism. However, new discoveries that the trigger point phenomena originate in the vicinity of dysfunctional endplates[11,12] puts an end to the previous claim. Melzack, in a subsequent article, defines acupuncture and trigger point dry needling as two distinctively different approaches.[13] Despite the similarities in terms of location between acupuncture points and trigger points, the objective clinician and researcher must recognize their distinct differences. These differences define acupuncture points and trigger points as two completely different clinical entities with possible overlaps.[5,14]

There are foundational and pathophysiological differences between trigger points and acupuncture points. Classical acupuncture points are identified as precise points along meridians defined by ancient Chinese documents.[9] An exception to that is extrameridian and "achi" points. Conversely, myofascial trigger points may be found anywhere within a muscle belly, and there is evidence that their pathophysiological mechanism resides in dysfunctional endplates.[12] Scientific merit requires that we are clear in our distinction between a trigger point and an acupuncture point.

Table 2-1

Differences Between Acupuncture and Trigger Point Dry Needling

	Trigger Point Dry Needling	Acupuncture
Pathophysiological Mechanism	Trigger points can be found anywhere in the muscle and originate in the vicinity of dysfunctional endplates[12]	Acupuncture points are found in precise locations identified by specific meridians[8,9] (except extra-meridian and achi points)
Clinical Application	Used for the assessment and treatment of myofascial pain syndrome due to myofascial trigger points[14-17]	Used for the diagnosis and treatment of several pathological conditions, including visceral and systemic dysfunction[7,8,18,19]
Physiological Response	Pain reduction established by inactivating a trigger point, thus eliminating the nociceptive focus of the muscle[12]	Pain relief achieved through release of endorphins;[2] results in balance of the body's energy levels[7]
Point Selection	Specifically defined essential and confirmatory criteria including a palpable taut band, nodularity, limited range of motion, referred pain pattern, local twitch response[12]	Selection of points is predetermined through the meridian-channel system[7-9] (except extra-meridian and achi points)
Needling Technique	One needle inserted in the trigger point, causing a local twitch response[4,20]	More than one needle is usually necessary[8,9]
Follow-Up Treatment	Application of myofascial stretching exercises are absolutely necessary to restore the proper length of the muscle and the correct muscle and joint mechanics[14,21]	Nothing similar is required
Clinical Requirements	Requires knowledge of the anatomy of the area, muscle and joint kinesiology and biomechanics, trigger point diagnostic techniques, and methods of needle application; applied by MDs and PTs	Requires knowledge of the entire diagnostic acupuncture system, including meridians and yin-yang principles; applied by licensed acupuncturists

As previously mentioned, a very effective clinical intervention for the treatment of myofascial pain syndrome is trigger point dry needling. While this intervention utilizes an acupuncture needle, it is distinctly different from acupuncture both in the rationale and its means of application.[5,14] It is important to understand that these two approaches are very different and require different training for their clinical application. Trigger point dry needling is practiced by properly trained medical doctors and physical therapists (when state laws and regulations permit). Table 2-1 describes some of the differences between trigger point dry needling and acupuncture.

REVIEW QUESTIONS

1. Myofascial trigger point therapy is identical to acupuncture treatment.
   True   (False)

2. Belgrade supports that tender points are acupuncture points and can often be chosen for therapy.
   (True)   False

3. Melzack et al found a ___71___ % correlation between trigger points and acupuncture points for the treatment of pain.

4. Melzack's contention is that trigger points and acupuncture points may have the same neural mechanism.
   (True)   False

5. Acupuncture and dry needling are two distinctly different techniques.
   (True)   False

6. Classical acupuncture points are identified as precise points along meridians defined by ancient Chinese documents.
   (True)   False

7. Myofascial trigger points may be in the tendon only and there is evidence that their pathophysiological mechanism resides in dysfunctional endplates.
   True   (False)

REFERENCES

1. Belgrade MJ. In response to the position paper of the NCAHF on acupuncture. *Clin J Pain.* 1992;8:183-4.

2. Belgrade MJ. Two decades after ping-pong diplomacy: is there a role for acupuncture in American pain medicine? *APS J.* 1994;3(2):73-83.

3. Lucente MM Jr, Belgrade MJ. Acupuncture and the law: a rebuttal. *N Engl J Med.* 1982;306:1115-6.

4. Hong CZ. Lidocaine injection versus dry needling to myofascial trigger point. The importance of the local twitch response. *Am J Phys Med Rehabil.* 1994;73:256-63.

5. Kostopoulos D, Rizopoulos K. Trigger point needling: PTs respond to education department's ruling on dry needling of trigger points. *Empire State Physical Therapy.* 1991:12-13.

6. Lewit K. The needle effect in the relief of myofascial pain. *Pain.* 1979;6:83-90.

7. Ellis A, Wiseman N, Boss K. *Fundamentals of Chinese Acupuncture.* Brookline, Mass: Paradigm Publications; 1991.

8. O'Connor J, Bensky D. *Acupuncture: A Comprehensive Text. Shanghai College Of Traditional Medicine.* Seattle, Wash: Eastland Press, Inc; 1981.

9. Stux G, Pomeranz B. *Acupuncture Textbook and Atlas.* New York: Springer-Verlag; 1987.

10. Melzack R, Stillwell DM, Fox EJ. Trigger points and acupuncture points for pain: correlations and implications. *Pain.* 1977;3:3-23.

11. Hong CZ, Simons DG. Pathophysiologic and electrophysiologic mechanisms of myofascial trigger points. *Arch Phys Med Rehabil.* 1998;79:863-72.

12. Travell JG, Simons DG, Simons LS. *Myofascial Pain and Dysfunction: The Trigger Point Manual—Upper Half of Body.* Baltimore, Md: Williams & Wilkins; 1999.

13. Melzack R. Myofascial trigger points: relation to acupuncture and mechanisms of pain. *Arch Phys Med Rehabil.* 1981;62:114-7.

14. Kostopoulos D, Rizopoulos K. Trigger point and myofascial therapy. *Advance for Physical Therapists.* 1998:25-28.

15. Simons DG. Examining for myofascial trigger points. *Arch Phys Med Rehabil.* 1993;74:676-7.

16. Talaat AM, el-Dibany MM, el-Garf A. Physical therapy in the management of myofascial pain dysfunction syndrome. *Ann Otol Rhinol Laryngol.* 1986;95:225-8.

17. Travell JG, Rinzler S. The myofascial genesis of pain. *Postgrad Med.* 1952;11:425-434.

18. Dumitru D. *Electrodiagnostic Medicine.* Philadelphia, Pa: Hanley & Belfus Inc; 1995.

19. Serizawa K. *Tsubo Vital Points for Oriental Therapy.* Tokyo: Japan Publications; 1976.

20. Fricton JR, Auvinen MD, Dykstra D, Schiffman E. Myofascial pain syndrome: electromyographic changes associated with local twitch response. *Arch Phys Med Rehabil.* 1985;66:314-7.

21. Kostopoulos D, Rizopoulos K, Brown A. Shin splint pain: the runner's nemesis. *Advance for Physical Therapists.* 1999:33-34.

Chapter 3

MUSCLE-NERVE PHYSIOLOGY AND CONTRACTION

THE MUSCLE

Skeletal muscle is a collection of muscle cells (muscle fibers). The number of muscle fibers depends on the size of the muscle and can vary from a few hundred to several thousand fibers. The entire muscle is covered and protected by connective fascial tissue, which is continuous with the connective tissue that surrounds each muscle fiber, tendon, bone, nerve, and vessel (Figure 3-1). The muscle is further divided into several muscle fascicles; each fascicle contains approximately 100 muscle fibers. Each fiber has a diameter of 50 to 100 µm (micrometers), a length of 2 to 6 cm (centimeters), and contains more than 1000 to 2000 myofibrils, which further consist of a chain of sarcomeres.[1] Each myofibril consists of several types of proteins (Figure 3-2).

CONTRACTILE PROTEINS

Actin[2,3] is the protein that makes up the thin filament of muscle fiber. Single molecules of G-actin (globular actin) polymerize together to form long chains of F-actin (fiber actin). Double-twisted helix-like strands of two F-actin polymers create the thin filaments of the myofibril.

Myosin[2,3] is a protein that consists of a single tail attached to two head portions, each of which extends out from the tail through an arm. One myosin filament contains 200 to 250 of these single-tail, two-headed molecules that together form a thick filament.[1] Each myosin head has two binding sites: a nucleotide binding site for binding with adenosine triphosphate (ATP) or adenosine diphosphate (ADP) and another site to bind with actin.

REGULATORY PROTEINS

Tropomyosin[2,3] is an elongated protein polymer that covers the actin filaments. Tropomyosin has an "on-off" switch, which is regulated by troponin. When tropomyosin is in the "off" position, it partially blocks the myosin-actin binding site and does not allow a power stroke to be completed during the muscle contraction. (Power stroke is defined as the translocation of the thin filaments toward the M-line of the sarcomere.) When tropomyosin is in the "on" position, it uncovers the remaining myosin-actin binding site to allow a complete interaction of the actin and myosin filaments, and, thus, a power stroke can be completed.

Troponin[2,3] consists of three globular proteins: troponin I, T, and C, which are attached to the tropomyosin filament at regular intervals. Troponin I binds strongly to actin; troponin T is attached to tropomyosin; and troponin-C binds with Ca^{2+}, causing a conformational change in the shape of the tropomyosin molecule. This turns the tropomyosin switch "on" to allow the interaction between actin and myosin filaments.

ACCESSORY PROTEINS

Titin[1,2] is a large elastic protein molecule that stabilizes the position of the contractile filaments and helps a stretched muscle return to its resting length.

Nebulin[1,2] is a large inelastic protein molecule that helps to maintain the structural framework of the sarcomere (see below), especially by playing a role in the proper alignment of the actin filaments.

SARCOMERE

Individual myofibrils consist of longitudinally repeated cylindrical units, called sarcomeres (Figure 3-3). Each sarcomere consists of thick and thin interdigitated filaments,

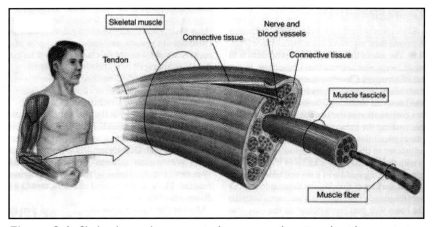

Figure 3-1. Skeletal muscle: anatomical summary (reprinted with permission from Silverthorn D. *Human Physiology: An Integrated Approach.* Upper Saddle River, NJ: Prentice Hall; 1998).

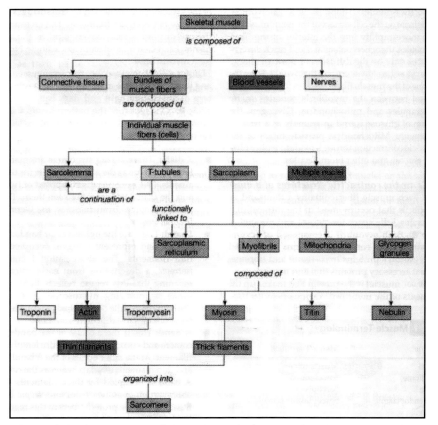

Figure 3-2. Composition of skeletal muscle (reprinted with permission from Silverthorn D. *Human Physiology: An Integrated Approach.* Upper Saddle River, NJ: Prentice Hall; 1998).

giving the myofibrils their characteristic alternate light and dark bands, which are bound by Z disks. Z disks are made of proteins and serve as attachments to the thin filaments. Each sarcomere includes two Z disks and thin filaments found between them. The sarcomere is the functional unit of length in skeletal muscle. The length of the sarcomere varies, however its physiological range is 1.5 to 3.5 mm. A 4-cm long muscle fiber at rest would have 20,000 sarcomeres in series.[2] The light band consists only of thin actin filaments and is called the I-band. The area of the sarcomere occupied by the thick myosin filaments is called the A-band. The presence of only an A-band in the sarcomere indicates maximum shortening and, therefore, complete overlap of the myofilaments.

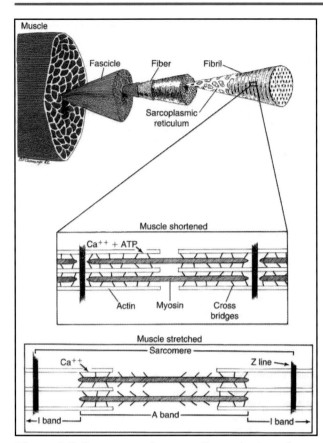

Figure 3-3. Structure and contractile mechanism of normal skeletal muscle (reprinted with permission from Travell JG, Simons DG, Simons LS. *Myofascial Pain and Dysfunction: The Trigger Point Manual—Upper Half of Body.* Baltimore, Md: Williams & Wilkins; 1999).

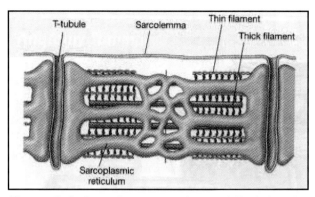

Figure 3-4. Sarcoplasmic reticulum and T-tubules: the sarcoplasmic reticulum wraps around each myofibril. The T-tubule system is closely associated with the sarcoplasmic reticulum (reprinted with permission from Silverthorn D. *Human Physiology: An Integrated Approach.* Upper Saddle River, NJ: Prentice Hall; 1998).

SARCOPLASMIC RETICULUM

The sarcoplasmic reticulum2,3 (Figure 3-4) is a tubular type of network that extends through the entire muscle. Longitudinal sarcoplasmic tubules end in a relatively large terminal cisternae at either end of the sarcomere. Two terminal cisternae in association with one T-tubule form a triad.1 Although these three structures are in very close association, there is no known connecting mechanism among them. The triad is critically positioned next to the part of the muscle fiber that produces the necessary forces for the contraction (Figure 3-5). The T-tubule plays an important role in conducting an action potential deep into the muscle. The role of the sarcoplasmic reticulum is to store Ca2+, which is necessary for the muscle contraction.

NERVOUS SYSTEM

The main job of the motor nervous system is to control and coordinate the function of the contractile elements in all the muscles simultaneously so that the correct tension is applied to the skeleton to produce the desired movement.[2]

The motor neuron is considered the functional unit of the motor nervous system.[4] The cell bodies of the motor neurons lie clustered into a motor nucleus within the ventral part of the spinal cord. The axon of each motor neuron exits the spinal cord through a ventral root (or through a cranial nerve from the brainstem) and divides into smaller branches of peripheral nerves until it enters into the muscle that is controlled by that nerve. When a large myelinated motor axon approaches a muscle fiber, it divides into multiple nerve twigs that run along the muscle's surface for short distances before ending. The region of a single muscle fiber lying under a nerve twig is called the motor endplate.

The cell body of an α-motoneuron, its axon, the endplates, and the muscle fibers innervated by that α-motoneuron comprise a motor unit[4] (Figure 3-6). In 98% of normal muscles, each muscle fiber receives its nerve supply from one motor endplate and, therefore, only one motor neuron. Exceptions to that are very long muscles, such as the sartorius.[4] One motor unit can supply hundreds of muscle fibers. Large muscles that perform gross motor activities have a high terminal innervation ratio (ratio of muscle fibers innervated by one nerve).[4] Muscles responsible for fine motor control, such as extraocular muscles, have a very low terminal innervation ratio—sometimes 1:1.

The end portion of the nerve, the axon terminal, is not in actual contact with the muscle fiber but separated by a distance of about 50 to 75 nm, called a synaptic cleft.

The terminal portion of each axon contains neurotubules, neurofilaments, mitochondria, and synaptic vesicles. The latter contain the neurotransmitter acetyl-

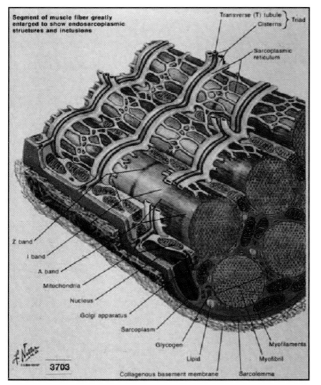

Figure 3-5. The triad consists of two cisterns and a transverse (T) tubule. (© 1994. ICON Learning Systems, LLC, a subsidiary of Havas MediMedia USA Inc. Reprinted with permission from ICON Learning Systems, LLC, illustrated by Frank H. Netter, MD. All rights reserved).

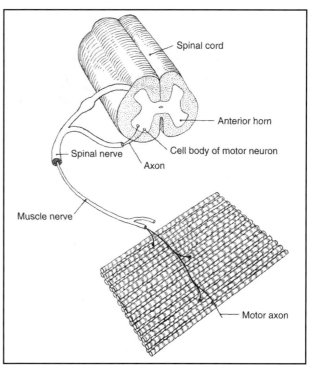

Figure 3-6. A motor unit consists of an α-motoneuron, its axon, an endplate, and the muscle fibers innervated by that α-motoneuron (reprinted with permission from Travell JG, Simons DG, Simons LS. *Myofascial Pain and Dysfunction: The Trigger Point Manual—Upper Half of Body.* Baltimore, Md: Williams & Wilkins; 1999).

choline (ACh). At rest, there is a spontaneous and random release of synaptic vesicles and ACh in the neuromuscular junction. This occurs as a result of the resting level of Ca^{2+} in the axon terminal, which is involved in the functioning of mitochondria.[4,5] Because of the presence of acetylcholinesterase (AChE) enzyme molecules, most of the released ACh hydrolyzes to choline and acetate. The remaining small quantity of the ACh is free to bind with its receptor, causing a small postsynaptic membrane depolarization, which is reflected electrophysiologically as a miniature endplate potential[4,6] (Figure 3-7).

MECHANISM OF MUSCLE CONTRACTION

In the early 1900s when scientists observed the properties of shortening and lengthening of muscle, they supported the idea that muscles were made up of molecules that curl up into shortened positions when active, then return to their resting length when relaxed. However, in 1954, Huxley and Niedeigerke proposed the "sliding filament theory of contraction."[2] According to this theory, in a contracting muscle, adjacent thick and thin filaments slide past each other, propelled by cyclical interactions

between the myosin heads of the thick filaments and binding sites on the actin of the adjacent thin filaments.[2] After an action potential is created, it travels down the myelinated nerve through saltatory conduction (jumping from node to Ranvier's node to node to Ranvier's node) with a speed up to 100 m/sec.[4,7] As the action potential nears the unmyelinated, small-diameter axon terminals, it slows down to 10 to 20 m/sec. When the action potential depolarizes, the terminal axon sodium and Ca^{2+} conductance increases, and Ca^{2+} ions are permitted to enter the terminal axon through the opening of voltage-gated Ca^{2+} channels at the active zone.[2] Presence of Ca^{2+} in the terminal axon will facilitate fusion of the ACh vesicles with the presynaptic membrane and release of large amounts of ACh in the synaptic cleft (see Figure 3-7). ACh binds to nicotinic cholinergic receptors that allow Na+ and K+ to cross the sarcolemma. As the Na+ influx is much greater than the K+ efflux, the transmembrane potential at the area of the endplate reverses (endplate potential) by as much as 75 mV (millivolts), depolarizing the adjacent muscle membrane.[4]

The action potential that moves across the membrane and down to the T-tubules is responsible for Ca^{2+} release from the sarcoplasmic reticulum.

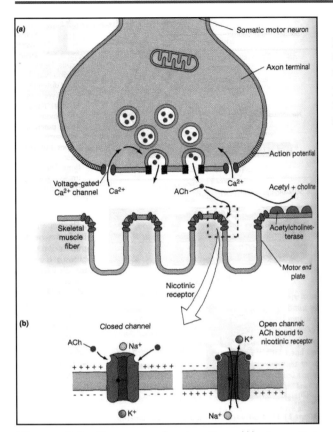

Figure 3-7. Neuromuscular junction: (A) an action potential opens voltage-gated Ca^{2+} channels in the axon terminal. Calcium ions enter the terminal, triggering exocytosis of synaptic vesicles. ACh in the synaptic cleft can combine with a nicotinic receptor on the motor endplate or be metabolized by AChE to acetyl and choline. (B) The nicotinic cholinergic receptor binds two ACh molecules, opening a nonspecific monovalent cation channel. Sodium ion influx exceeds K^+ efflux, and the muscle fiber depolarizes (reprinted with permission from Silverthorn D. *Human Physiology: An Integrated Approach.* Upper Saddle River, NJ: Prentice Hall; 1998).

When cytosolic Ca^{2+} levels increase, Ca^{2+} binds to troponin. The binding of Ca^{2+} to the troponin changes the shape of the associated tropomyosin, which uncovers the remainder of the myosin-binding site and allows the power stroke to be completed and move to the next actin molecule (Figures 3-8 and 3-9). Following is the sequence:[2]

* When the muscle is at rest, there is no binding between the troponin molecule and Ca^{2+}; therefore, tropomyosin will allow only partial interaction between actin and myosin. The myosin heads are in a "cocked" position with bound adenosine diphosphate (ADP).

* Upon the presence of an action potential and the release of ionized Ca^{2+} from the sarcoplasmic reticulum, Ca^{2+} binds with troponin, which causes a conformational change in the associated tropomyosin. This action causes exposure of the actin-binding site, allowing the myosin heads to attach and form "cross bridges" between actin and myosin filaments. Myosin heads are at a 90-degree angle.

* Myosin heads rotate to form a 45-degree angle, causing a further sliding action between actin and myosin filaments. This creates shortening of the muscle fiber. At this point, ADP is detached from the myosin.

* At the end of the cross bridge power stroke, a new molecule of adenosine triphosphate (ATP) binds to the myosin head at the nucleotide-binding site.

* ATP hydrolyzes to ADP and inorganic phosphate. The chemical energy released is used to recock the myosin head to a new binding site and, thus, another power stroke.

This process continuously repeats during a muscle contraction. In a normal muscle, the free Ca^{2+} is quickly pumped back into the sarcoplasmic reticulum. The absence of Ca^{2+} terminates the contractile activity and the muscle relaxes. Presence of ATP is crucial as an energy source for this process. When ATP supplies are exhausted, as in the state after death, muscles are unable to bind more ATP and thus remain in a tightly bound state called *rigor mortis*. In this state, the muscles form immovable cross bridges.

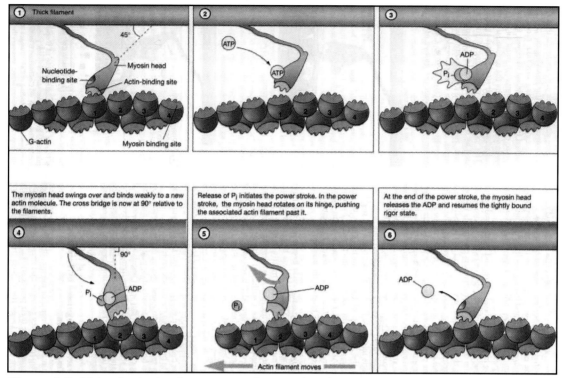

Figure 3-8. Molecular basis of contraction (reprinted with permission from Silverthorn D. *Human Physiology: An Integrated Approach.* Upper Saddle River, NJ: Prentice Hall; 1998).

REVIEW QUESTIONS

1. Actin and myosin are regulatory proteins.
   True   False

2. One myosin filament contains 200 to 250 single-tail, two-headed molecules that jointly form a thin filament.
   True   False

3. Titin and nebulin are considered proteins.
   True   False

4. Nebulin helps to maintain the structural framework of the sarcomere, especially by playing a role in the proper alignment of the actin filaments.
   True   False

5. The sarcomere is considered the functional unit of length in skeletal muscle.
   True   False

6. The light band consists only of ___Actin___ filaments and is called an I-band.

7. The area of the sarcomere occupied by the thick myosin filaments is called an A-band.
   True   False

8. The presence of only an A-band and absence of an I-band in the sarcomere indicates maximum lengthening of the myofilaments.
   True   False

9. Two terminal cisternae in association with one T-tubule form a _____.

10. The primary role of the sarcoplasmic reticulum is to store potassium (K) that is necessary for the muscle contraction.
    True   False

11. The region of a single muscle fiber lying under a nerve twig is defined as the _____

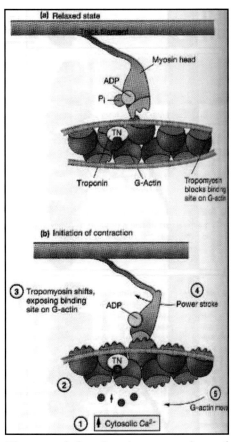

Figure 3-9. Regulatory role of tropomyosin and troponin (reprinted with permission from Silverthorn D. *Human Physiology: An Integrated Approach.* Upper Saddle River, NJ: Prentice Hall; 1998).

REFERENCES

1. Silverthorn D. *Human Physiology: An Integrated Approach.* Upper Saddle River, NJ: Prentice Hall; 1998.
2. Kandel E, Schartz J, Jessell TM. *Principles of Neural Science.* 4th ed. New York: McGraw-Hill; 2000.
3. Fawcett D. *A Textbook of Histology.* Philadelphia, Pa: WB Saunders; 1986.
4. Dumitru D. *Electrodiagnostic Medicine.* Philadelphia, Pa: Hanley & Belfus Inc; 1995.
5. Alnaes E, Rahamimoff R. On the role of mitochondria in transmitter release from motor nerve terminals. *J Physiol.* 1975;285-306.
6. Fatt P, Katz B. Spontaneous subthreshold activity of motor nerve endings. *J Physiol.* 1952;109-128.
7. Kimura J. *Electrodiagnosis in Diseases of Nerve and Muscle.* Philadelphia, Pa: FA Davis; 1989.

12. The cell body of an α-motoneuron, its axon, the endplates, and the muscle fibers innervated by that α-motoneuron comprise a ___motorunit___

13. Huxley and Niedeigerke proposed the "sliding filament theory of contraction."
    True   False

14. Presence of Ca^{2+} in the terminal axon will facilitate fusion of the ACh vesicles with the presynaptic membrane and release of an electric impulse in the synaptic cleft.
    True   False

15. ATP is used as an energy source for the muscle contraction.
    True   False

Chapter 4

PATHOGENESIS OF MYOFASCIAL TRIGGER POINTS

To enhance uniformity and better understand a myofascial trigger point, we will adopt the definition of a trigger point as described by Travell and Simons.

DEFINITION

Travell and Simons[1,2] define a myofascial trigger point as "...a hyperirritable spot in skeletal muscle that is associated with a hypersensitive palpable nodule in a taut band. The spot is painful on compression and can give rise to characteristic referred pain, referred tenderness, motor dysfunction, and autonomic phenomena." Myofascial trigger points may decrease muscle flexibility, produce muscle weakness, and distort proprioception. Other types of trigger points include cutaneous, fascial, ligamentus, and periosteal trigger points, which are not the focus of this book.

PATHOPHYSIOLOGY OF A TRIGGER POINT

There are various hypotheses regarding the pathogenesis and pathophysiology of a myofascial trigger point. The most important ones are:

1. *Muscle spindle hypothesis* introduced by Hubbard and Berkoff.[3] According to them, abnormal muscle spindles are responsible for the production of abnormal electrophysiological signals, such as spontaneous electrical activity and spikes detected in the proximity of a trigger point. Therefore, an abnormal muscle spindle could play an important role in the pathogenesis of the trigger point. Well-documented recent studies[4,5] clearly demonstrate that these abnormal electrophysiological signals are detectable only in the vicinity of a trigger point and somewhat in the endplate zone. Muscle spindles are scattered throughout the entire muscle, including areas where there is no abnormal electromyographic (EMG) activity, something that discounts Hubbard and Berkoff's hypothesis. In addition, one of the clinically effective treatments for myofascial trigger points is injection of botulinum A toxin.[6-9] This toxin directly affects the neuromuscular junction by denervating the cell of the injected muscle on the muscle spindle. Therefore, the pathophysiological mechanism of myofascial trigger points should be one that includes the effects of an abnormal endplate, neuromuscular junction, or abnormal postsynaptic membrane.

The authors of this book believe that the muscle spindle plays a contributory role in the continuous presence of trigger points in the muscle by creating tonic disturbances and spasm on the involved muscle (see Figure 4-2). In addition, due to the muscle imbalance present in a region where one or more muscles are myofascially involved, muscle spindles may be responsible for spasm in adjacent muscles with no apparent trigger points present. Abnormal joint mechanics in the presence of a muscle imbalance will create unfamiliar compensatory movements of the body with abnormal firing and contraction rates. This process may affect the intrafusal fibers and impede the normal function of a muscle spindle by resetting its sensitivity at a higher level.[10,11] This may account for the sensation of heightened muscle tension.[10] Treatments, such as *strain-counter strain* and *postisometric relaxation* that "reset" the mechanism of the muscle spindle are very effective and can be used in conjunction with the mainstream treatments for myofascial trigger points.

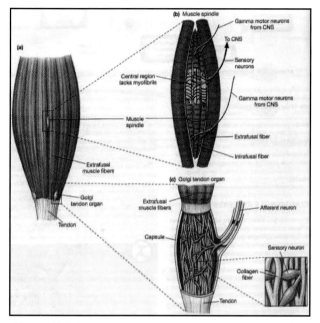

Figure 4-1. Muscle sensory receptors. The central region of the muscle spindle (b) lacks myofibrils and cannot contract. Sensory nerve endings wrap around the central region and fire when the central section of the muscle spindle stretches. The ends of the muscle spindle contain myofibrils that contract in response to commands carried by gamma motor neurons (reprinted with permission from Silverthorn D. *Human Physiology: An Integrated Approach.* Upper Saddle River, NJ: Prentice Hall; 1998).

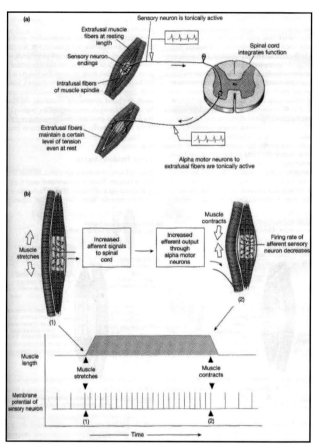

Figure 4-2. Muscle spindle function. (a) When a muscle is at its resting length, the muscle spindle is slightly stretched and its associated sensory neuron shows tonic activity. As a result of tonic reflex activity, the associated muscle maintains a certain level of tension or tone, even at rest. (b) If a muscle is stretched, its muscle spindles are also stretched. This stretching increases the firing rate of the spindle afferents, and the muscle contracts. Contraction relieves the stretch on the spindle and acts as negative feedback to diminish the reflex (reprinted with permission from Silverthorn D. *Human Physiology: An Integrated Approach.* Upper Saddle River, NJ: Prentice Hall; 1998).

2. *Hypothesis of neuropathic process* introduced by Gunn.[12-14] He proposed that when the nerve that innervates the affected muscle is involved in a neuropathic process it may cause hypersensitivity and myofascial trigger points. It is the opinion of the authors of this book that neuropathic process of proximal or distal origin may have an effect in the neuromuscular junction and the endplate, and become a leading factor in the pathogenesis of myofascial trigger points.

3. The *scar tissue hypothesis* is derived from various histological studies identifying scar fibrous tissue in the vicinity of a severely damaged scar tissue. Although a chronic unresolved myofascial trigger point syndrome can lead to scar tissue formation, scar tissue is not a necessary histologic finding in the area of a trigger point or at the area of a contraction knot.[15]

4. *Hypothesis of dysfunctional endplates and energy crisis,* introduced by Simons,[1,16] is the most recent and well-documented theory regarding the creation of trigger points. This theory, along with our own understanding regarding the pathophysiology of trigger points, will be presented here.

MECHANISM OF INJURY

Overstretching, overshortening, or overloading a muscle, especially in a prolonged fashion, may cause a microtrauma. When a muscle becomes overstretched, overshortened, or overloaded, part of the muscle fiber may be destroyed through rupture of the muscle cell membrane (sarcolemma) (Figure 4-3).[10]

Microtrauma can be the result of:

* Repetitive movement: we very often see presence of myofascial trigger points in individuals suffering from repetitive strain injuries.

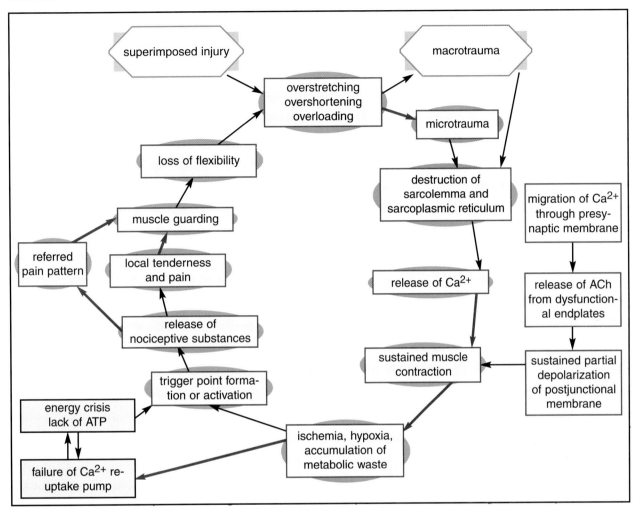

Figure 4-3. Mechanism of injury and activation of myofascial trigger points.

the body with sufficient blood circulation would remove the Ca^{2+} from the area and the muscle would return to its resting position. However, according to Simons and Hong,[1,16] a possible local dysfunction of the endplate (dysfunctional endplate) will produce a continuous and excessive release of ACh in the synaptic cleft, constantly depolarizing the postjunctional membrane. The presence of AChE in the synaptic cleft is not adequate to hydrolyze the larger quantities of released ACh.

It is the opinion of the authors that irritation and disturbance of the presynaptic membrane will open more frequently than normal voltage-gated Ca^{2+} channels. At the same time, large quantities of free-floating Ca^{2+} exist in the area of the synaptic cleft that have been released by the destruction of the sarcoplasmic reticulum. This Ca^{2+} will enter the presynaptic membrane, causing a facilitation of the synaptic vesicles to attach to the presynaptic membrane and diffuse ACh across the synaptic cleft. Therefore, a maximum and sustained contractile activity of the sarcomeres will be present. This sustained muscle

cause histologic changes and trigger point formation or reactivation of a previously active trigger point that is currently latent.

Severe local hypoxia and a tissue energy crisis will lead to the release of substances that can sensitize muscle nociceptors, causing pain (Figure 4-4). Release of bradykinin (cleaved from plasma proteins), prostaglandins (synthesized from endothelial cells), and histamine (released from mast cells) will cause sensitization effects.[22]

In addition to the local tenderness and nociception, a referred pain pattern may develop in distal parts of the body. Further shortening of the sarcomere will cause a decrease in the length of the muscle (Figure 4-5). This pathophysiological shortening of the muscle, along with muscle guarding due to pain, will lead to further loss of flexibility, which may affect proper joint mechanics. The muscles, as well as the adjacent structures, are more vulnerable to a possible superimposed injury leading to a macrotrauma. This is very evident in individuals who have initial symptoms explained as a myofascial trigger

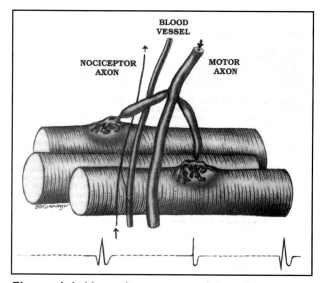

Figure 4-4. Mammalian motor endplates. Notice that blood vessels and nociceptor axons are found near the motor endplates. These axons may transmit afferent nociceptive signals stimulated by various sensitizing substances released in the area (reprinted with permission from Salpeter MM. *The Vertebrate Neuromuscular Junction.* New York: Alan R Liss, Inc; 1987).

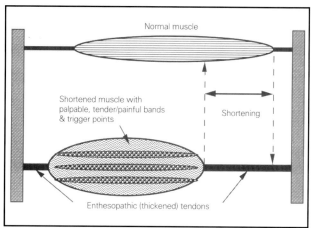

Figure 4-5. Shortening of muscle at the presence of myofascial trigger point (reprinted with permission from Gunn C. *Treating Myofascial Pain: Intramuscular Stimulation (IMS) for Myofascial Pain Syndromes of Neuropathic Origin.* Seattle, Wash: University of Washington; 1989).

point syndrome (possible microtrauma) that is never treated and becomes the underlying cause of a future injury that is greater in magnitude (macrotrauma).

Many sports injuries are the result of a superimposed trauma by a previously myofascially involved muscle. For example, a baseball pitcher suffering from mild to moderate shoulder pain as a result of tightening and the presence of myofascial trigger points in the subscapularis and infraspinatus muscles—if one neglects to correctly treat the shoulder and restore proper shoulder mechanics, this pre-existing injury may result in a macrotrauma, such as concentric macrotrauma of the subscapularis muscle along with an eccentric macrotrauma of the infraspinatus muscle, including a possible tear.

REVIEW QUESTIONS

1. Myofascial trigger points have no effect on muscle flexibility.
    True   *False*

2. According to the muscle spindle hypothesis, abnormal muscle spindles are responsible for the production of abnormal electrophysiological signals such as spontaneous electrical activity and spikes detected in the proximity of a trigger point.
    True   False

3. The hypothesis of neuropathic process was first introduced by Hubbard.
    True   *False*

4. According to this text, microtrauma can be the result of: repeditiue, high velocity, and stress positing   movements

5. According to Simons and Hong,[4,5] a dysfunctional endplate can produce a continuous and excessive release of ACh in the synaptic cleft that will depolarize the postjunctional membrane in a constant fashion.
    True   False

6. One of the points that challenged the muscle spindle hypothesis is:
    A. That trigger points are hypersensitive nodular entities.
    B. That muscle spindles are scattered within a muscle, while trigger points are usually found near or at the endplate zone.
    C. That muscle spindles will be deactivated when injecting botulinum A toxin and therefore cannot be the cause of a trigger point.
    D. That muscle spindles reveal abnormal electromyographic signals.

REFERENCES

1. Travell JG, Simons DG, Simons LS. *Myofascial Pain and Dysfunction: The Trigger Point Manual—Upper Half of Body.* Baltimore, Md: Williams & Wilkins; 1999.

2. Travell JG, Simons DG. *Myofascial Pain and Dysfunction: The Trigger Point Manual.* Vol 1. Baltimore, Md: Williams & Wilkins; 1983.

3. Hubbard DR, Berkoff GM. Myofascial trigger points show spontaneous needle EMG activity. *Spine.* 1993;18:1803-7.

4. Simons D, Hong C, Simons LS. Nature of myofascial trigger points, active loci. *Journal of Musculoskeletal Pain.* 1995;3(1Suppl):62.

5. Simons D, Hong C, Simons LS. Prevalence of spontaneous electrical activity at trigger spots and control sites in rabbit muscle. *Journal of Musculoskeletal Pain.* 1995;3(1):35-48.

6. Acquadro MA, Borodic GE. Treatment of myofascial pain with botulinum A toxin. *Anesthesiology.* 1994;80:705-6.

7. Cheshire WP, Abashian SW, Mann JD. Botulinum toxin in the treatment of myofascial pain syndrome. *Pain.* 1994;59:65-9.

8. Diaz JH, Gould HJ III. Management of post-thoracotomy pseudoangina and myofascial pain with botulinum toxin. *Anesthesiology.* 1999;91:877-9.

9. Porta M. A comparative trial of botulinum toxin type A and methylprednisolone for the treatment of myofascial pain syndrome and pain from chronic muscle spasm. *Pain.* 2000;85:101-5.

10. Bennett R. *Advances in Pain Research and Therapy: Myofascial Pain Syndromes and the Fibromyalgia Syndrome: A Comparative Analysis.* New York: Raven Press; 1990;17:43-65.

11. Dorko LB. Shallow dive: essays on the craft of manual care. *Ockham's Razor.* 20-21.

12. Gunn CC. Fibromyalgia—what have we created? (Wolfe 1993). *Pain.* 1995;60:349-50.

13. Gunn CC. Chronic pain: time for epidemiology. *J R Soc Med.* 1996;89:479-80.

14. Gunn C. *The Gunn Approach to the Treatment of Chronic Pain—Intramuscular Stimulation for Myofascial Pain of Radiculopathic Origin.* London: Churchill Livingstone; 1996.

15. Simons D, Stolov W. Microscopic features and transient contraction of palpable bands in canine muscle. *Am J Phys Med.* 1976;55:65-88.

16. Hong CZ, Simons DG. Pathophysiologic and electrophysiologic mechanisms of myofascial trigger points. *Arch Phys Med Rehabil.* 1998;79:863-72.

17. Pawl RP. Chronic neck syndromes: an update. *Compr Ther.* 1999;25:278-82.

18. Simons DG. Fibrositis/fibromyalgia: a form of myofascial trigger points? *Am J Med.* 1986;81:93-8.

19. Simons DG. Myofascial pain syndromes: where are we? where are we going? *Arch Phys Med Rehabil.* 1988;69:207-12.

20. Simons DG. Familial fibromyalgia and/or myofascial pain syndrome? *Arch Phys Med Rehabil.* 1990;71:258-9.

21. Simons DG. Reply to MI Weintraub. *Pain.* 1999;80:451-2.

22. Mense S, Simons D, Russell I. *Muscle Pain: Understanding its Nature, Diagnosis and Treatment.* Baltimore, Md: Lippincott Williams & Wilkins; 2001.

Chapter 5

CLINICAL SYMPTOMS AND PHYSICAL FINDINGS

Myofascial trigger points present various clinical symptoms that are identified by the clinician during the patient interview. During the patient examination, several physical findings may be elicited by the clinician.

CLINICAL SYMPTOMS

ONSET

Activation of myofascial trigger points are associated with some degree to microtrauma. This does not necessarily require a sudden high-velocity movement. A microtrauma may occur through a repetitive continuous motion or even through an overload of the muscle through a stress position (postural stresses, functional and structural asymmetries). Many times the patient will be able to identify the cause of the dysfunction, especially if it is related to a sudden high-velocity movement or if related to an unusual activity. Other times the patient will be able to identify just the pain symptom. In some cases, the patient will identify a previous injury or a past diagnosis as the cause of pain. The clinician must be careful, especially when the condition has a neuropathic origin. Central or peripheral nerve compression, especially when the degree of the compression is such that causes electrophysiologic changes, may facilitate activation of myofascial trigger points.

LOCAL PAIN

The patient will most frequently complain of referred pain and occasionally of pain, burning sensation, and tenderness on the involved muscle. Several nociceptive substances have been identified in the proximity of a myofascial trigger point. These include bradykinin, E-type prostaglandins, 5-hydroxytryptamine, and a higher concentration in hydrogen ions that decrease the pH. Nociceptor axons in the area are responsible for noxious stimuli (see Figure 4-4).

REFERRED PAIN PATTERN

Myofascial trigger points refer pain to distal or proximal locations in specific patterns that are characteristic for each muscle. Activation of a trigger point projects pain to a distant reference zone. This is called a referred pain pattern (RPP) and is one of the criteria used to identify the appropriate muscle to treat. It is important for the clinician to understand that utilizing the RPP as the only criterion to decide what muscle to treat will often lead to false treatment. There are additional factors involved in the decision that will be thoroughly discussed in subsequent chapters. In very few cases, the RPP may follow part of the same dermatome, myotome, or scleratome. However, this does not always occur. In general, RPPs are not segmental (Figure 5-1).

AUTONOMIC AND PROPRIOCEPTIVE DISTURBANCES

Disturbances of various autonomic functions, such as excessive sweating and salivation, may be present. Other autonomic phenomena, such as a positive pilomotor reflex (goose bumps) (Figure 5-2) or redness around the trigger point area, may exist. Distorted proprioception is very frequent. Dizziness, lack of balance, and tinnitus can be present in more severe and chronic cases. In addition, the proprioceptors of the sole, deep neck extensors, and

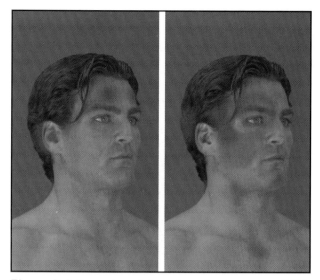

Figure 5-1. Examples of the referred pain pattern (RPP) of the sternocleidomastoid muscle. The trigger point refers pain to distal locations, as illustrated in these photographs, which is characteristic for this muscle.

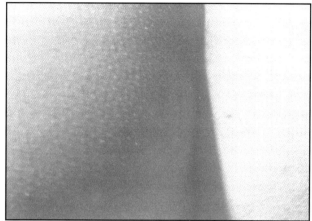

Figure 5-2. The pilomotor reflex is one of the autonomic disturbances that may be present near the area of a myofascial trigger point (reprinted with permission from Gunn C. *Treating Myofascial Pain: Intramuscular Stimulation (IMS) for Myofascial Pain Syndromes of Neuropathic Origin.* Seattle, Wash: University of Washington; 1989).

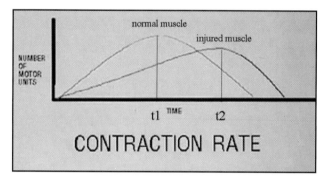

Figure 5-3. A slower contraction rate will create a slower recruitment of motor units.

the sacroiliac joint may be disturbed, causing an abnormal flow of proprioceptive input. The contraction rate (time of recruitment of the maximum number of motor units required for contraction) will slow down, making the neuromuscular function slower and exposing the muscle to danger of future injury (Figure 5-3).

EDEMA AND CELLULITE

Due to the decreased blood circulation and accumulation of the products of cellular metabolism, the area may develop local edema. This can be easily identified using the "matchstick test." Skin indentations produced by the acute instrument will remain for a prolonged period of time, indicating local edema (Figure 5-4). Presence of cellulite is not uncommon (Figure 5-5).

DERMATOMAL HAIR LOSS

In cases of myofascial trigger points present in the paraspinal muscle, Gunn[3] reported hair loss to the corresponding dermatome depending on the spinal level involved (Figure 5-6).

SLEEP DISTURBANCES

Patients will often complain of lack of sleep due to pain, numbness, burning sensation, or other disturbances. Patients usually assume an antalgic, temporarily comfortable position during the night that puts the muscle in a shortened position. This may cause further activation of myofascial trigger points (through overshortening) and further loss of flexibility.

PHYSICAL FINDINGS

TAUT BAND

The taut band includes those muscle fibers that are myofascially involved (Figure 5-7). Rubbing across these fibers gives a rope-like sensation. The myofascially involved fibers include local areas with overshortened sarcomeres as well as overstretched areas. The overshortened sarcomeres reflect the focus on and around the myofascial trigger point, while the overstretched ones represent the distant areas of the same muscle fibers. After the trigger point is resolved, the taut band may disappear.

TENDER AND PAINFUL NODULES

When palpating along the taut band, the entire area will demonstrate some tenderness; however, the locus

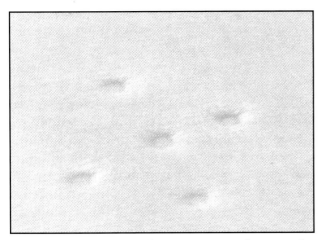

Figure 5-4. Edema may be present near the area of a myofascial trigger point due to circulatory problems (reprinted with permission from Gunn C. *Treating Myofascial Pain: Intramuscular Stimulation (IMS) for Myofascial Pain Syndromes of Neuropathic Origin.* Seattle, Wash: University of Washington; 1989).

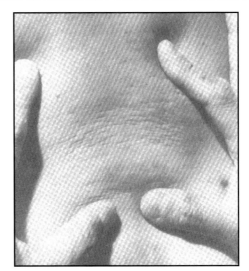

Figure 5-5. Cellulite may be present near the area of a myofascial trigger point (reprinted with permission from Gunn C. *Treating Myofascial Pain: Intramuscular Stimulation (IMS) for Myofascial Pain Syndromes of Neuro-pathic Origin.* Seattle, Wash: University of Washington; 1989).

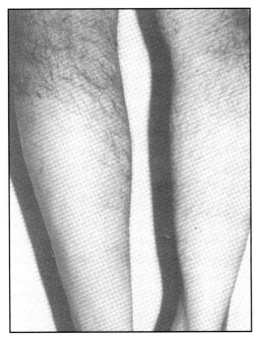

Figure 5-6. Dermatomal hair loss may be present in cases of myofascial trigger points in the paraspinal muscles (reprinted with permission from Gunn C. *Treating Myofascial Pain: Intramuscular Stimulation (IMS) for Myofascial Pain Syndromes of Neuropathic Origin.* Seattle, Wash: University of Washington; 1989).

PATIENT PAIN RECOGNITION

Ischemic compression or needle insertion on the myofascial trigger point may exhibit pain or other sensation that is recognizable by the patient as similar to the main symptom he or she experiences. Patient pain recognition is one of the essential criteria for the diagnosis of a myofascial trigger point.

LOCAL TWITCH RESPONSE

Local twitch response (LTR) is produced through a local depolarization of the muscle membrane of the myofascially involved fibers (taut band area). It can be elicited either through pincer snapping palpation across the taut band (see Figure 5-7) or through a needle insertion. LTR may have a therapeutic effect by causing metabolic changes in the area. Multiple LTRs are induced through the trigger point dry needling technique and seem to have a positive effect on the resolution of the myofascial trigger point. LTR through snapping palpation can be useful in the release of persistent, unresolved trigger points.

LIMITED RANGE OF MOTION

Due to the abnormal tension and tenderness present in the taut band, the myofascially involved muscle will exhibit limitation in range of motion, especially at the end range of movement. Muscle stiffness and tightness are very common, especially after hours of prolonged immobility, such as in the early morning hours.

directly on and around the myofascial trigger point will exhibit nodularity and exquisite pain. Progressively increasing pressure on the nodule will elicit the RPP and possibly the sign of patient pain recognition.

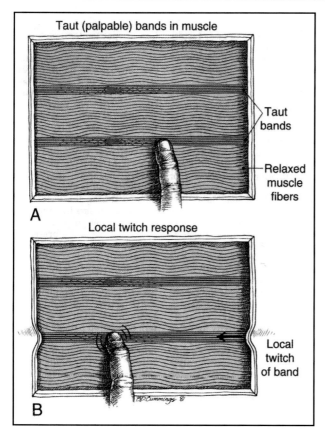

Taut (palpable) bands in muscle

Taut bands

Relaxed muscle fibers

A

Local twitch response

Local twitch of band

B

Figure 5-7. Palpation of a taut band. Rolling the band quickly under the fingertip (snapping palpation) at the trigger point often produces a local twitch response (reprinted with permission from Travell JG, Simons DG, Simons LS. *Myofascial Pain and Dysfunction: The Trigger Point Manual—Upper Half of Body.* Baltimore, Md: Williams & Wilkins; 1999).

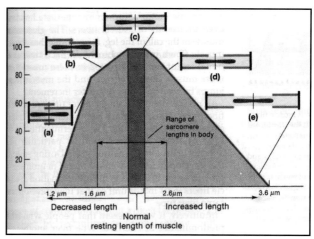

Figure 5-8. Length-tension relationships in contracting muscle. The graph shows the amount of tension generated by a muscle compared with its resting length before contraction begins. The inserts of the sarcomeres show the amount of overlap between thick and thin filaments at each resting muscle length. If the muscle is too long, the filaments in the sarcomere barely overlap and cannot form as many crossbridge links (e). If the muscle begins its contraction at a very short length, the sarcomere cannot shorten very much before the myosin filaments run into the Z disks at each end (a) (reprinted with permission from Silverthorn D. *Human Physiology: An Integrated Approach.* Upper Saddle River, NJ: Prentice Hall; 1998).

MUSCLE WEAKNESS

Muscle weakness is commonly seen in patients with myofascial trigger points, and there are various possible sources to account for it. Usually the manual muscle test will result in half to one grade lower in the involved muscle as compared to the rest of the uninvolved muscles of the same side or the muscles of the uninvolved side. The length-tension relationship curve (Figure 5-8) explains how overshortened sarcomeres allow the formation of a lesser number of cross bridges between actin and myosin filaments. This will result in a decrease in the tension that the muscle can possibly develop. It is clinically evident that application of myofascial trigger point therapy followed by myofascial stretching exercises can improve muscle strength by promoting lengthening of the sarcomeres and therefore creating the potential for formation of a larger number of cross bridges between the myofilaments. In addition, spasm of the myofascially involved

muscle will cause local ischemia resulting in decreased energy sources. This may affect muscle performance. Muscle guarding due to local or referred pain can produce antalgic movement and subsequently poor muscle performance. Research demonstrates that muscles with myofascial trigger points fatigue more rapidly and become exhausted sooner than normal muscles.[1,2] Muscle imbalances may develop, with various muscles prone to inhibition and therefore weakness, while others are prone to excitation and therefore tightness.

POSITIVE STRETCH SIGN

Positive stretch sign (PSS) is defined as any pain of mechanical or neural origin that develops in the joint during myofascial stretching. Passive or active stretching of a muscle with active myofascial trigger points, especially to the end of range, is inhibited. The increased tension of the taut bands will inhibit the muscle to extend to its full range and will affect proper joint mechanics. The resulting movement will be compromised, with altered and abnormal joint mechanics. This abnormal movement will create stresses to the joint, resulting in pain. When PSS is elicited during myofascial stretching, it is an indication that pushing through to further stretching could be harmful. Returning the muscle to its resting position and applying additional trigger point therapy (ischemic compression or other techniques) will further decrease the activity of the trigger point and will allow us to achieve a greater range of motion at this time.

Alternating back and forth between trigger point therapy and myofascial stretching exercise seems to be the most effective approach to treatment. PSS guides the clinician to decide on the extent of myofascial stretch that is appropriate at a given time (eg, treating a patient with a diagnosis of shoulder impingement and active myofascial trigger points on the subscapularis [SSC] muscle). After the application of ischemic compression to the SSC muscle, the clinician follows with the appropriate myofascial stretch. In this case, achieving full abduction of the shoulder is desired. At about 70 degrees of shoulder abduction, the patient complains of pain at the top of the acromion (impingement). This type of pain is defined as a PSS because it was developed during the stretching action of the treatment. Apparently, the pain has a mechanical origin and derives from improper joint mechanics of a myofascially involved tight SSC. Bringing the muscle back to a relaxed position and working further with ischemic compression on the trigger point will allow us to repeat the stretch without eliciting pain (PSS) until we reach 85 degrees of shoulder abduction. We continue back and forth, alternating between ischemic compression and stretching, several times, noticing that as the trigger point activity decreases we are able to achieve a further increase in the range of motion. To not pay attention to the PSS and stretch the muscle aggressively regardless of joint pain can be counterproductive to the treatment and harmful to the patient.

PSS should not be confused with local muscle soreness and tenderness from the referred pain pattern. If local muscle soreness develops, one may use the "spray and stretch" technique and continue within the patient's tolerance limit.

REVIEW QUESTIONS

1. A microtrauma may occur only through a high-velocity movement.
   True   False

2. The reason for local pain in the area of a trigger point is the presence of Ca^{2+}.
   True   False

3. Myofascial trigger points refer pain to distal or proximal locations in specific patterns characteristic for each muscle.
   True   False

4. Overstretched sarcomeres reflect the locus on and around the myofascial trigger point, while overshortened ones represent the distant areas of the same muscle fibers.
   True   False

5. Patient pain recognition and referred pain patterns have identical definitions.
   True   False

6. It is possible that patient pain recognition and referred pain patterns extend to exactly the same area.
   True   False

7. Local twitch response is produced through a local depolarization of the muscle membrane of the myofascially involved fibers.
   True   False

8. Presence of myofascial trigger points in a muscle has no effect on the range of motion, muscle strength, and flexibility.
   True   False

9. Pain of mechanical or neural origin that develops in the joint during myofascial stretching is defined as _positive stretch sign_

10. During the application of trigger point therapy (digital compression of the trigger point) the patient complains of pain and states "this feels like the kind of pain I usually have." Would you define this as:
    A. Positive stretch sign
    B. Patient pain recognition
    C. Referred pain pattern
    D. None of the above

11. During the application of myofascial stretching of the iliopsoas muscle, the patient complains of slight soreness in the anterior thigh by the insertion of the iliopsoas. According to the authors, this is a:
    A. Positive stretch sign. Stretching must stop. Do more digital compression and repeat stretching.
    B. Patient pain recognition. Stop treatment immediately.
    C. Pain due to muscle stretching. Use spray and stretch and continue within the patient's limits of tolerance.
    D. None of the above.

REFERENCES

1. Headley B. Assessing surface EMG. *Rehabilitation Management*. 1992;5:87-91.

2. Headley B. Evaluation and treatment of myofascial pain syndrome utilizing biofeedback. In: *Clinical EMG for Surface Recordings*. Nevada City, Nev: Clinical Resources; 1990:235-254.

3. Gunn CC. *Treating Myofascial Pain: Intramuscular Stimulation (IMS) for Myofascial Pain Syndromes of Neuropathic Origin*. Seattle, Wash: University of Washington; 1989.

Chapter 6

REFERRED PAIN PATTERN MECHANISMS

While there is no one specific mechanism clearly identified as responsible for the referred pain pattern of myofascial trigger points, there are various possible mechanisms that may share responsibility.

A pain stimulus to be perceived by the sensory cortex is transformed at least four times on at least four levels:

1. The receptor site converts the stimulus into a nerve impulse.
2. The spinal cord level.
3. The network structures between the spinal cord and the sensory cortex (thalamus).
4. The sensory cortex itself.

In 1969, Selzer and Spencer[1,2] postulated five different mechanisms to explain referred pain:

1. Peripheral branching of primary afferent axons: The brain misinterprets messages originating from nerve endings in one part of the body if originating from another part of the body.
2. Convergence-projection: A single nerve cell in the spinal cord receives nociceptive stimuli both by internal organs and by the skin and/or muscles. The sensory cortex cannot distinguish whether the information had a visceral or cutaneous origin and misinterprets the nociceptive signal.
3. Convergence-facilitation: Cutaneous sensory afferent activity; if insufficient quantity to excite the spinothalamic tract, it is facilitated by strong abnormal visceral afferent activity interpreted as pain.
4. Sympathetic nervous system activity: Sympathetic fibers release nociceptive substances (prostaglandins) that sensitize primary afferent nerve endings in the region of a trigger point.
5. Convergence or image projection at the supraspinal level: Convergence of pain pathways at a supraspinal, thalamic level.

Quintner and Cohen[3] challenge the premise that a myofascial trigger point gives rise to a referred pain pattern. They suggest that "all myofascial pain syndrome phenomena are better explained as secondary hyperalgesia of peripheral nerve origin."

Simons supports that one of the mechanisms responsible for referred pain is the peripheral sensitization of nociceptors.[4] The presence of bradykinin, E-type prostaglandins, and 5-hydroxytrimptamine near the active loci can create sensitization effects contributing to the referred pain mechanism. A recent study using the animal model of rabbit tissue demonstrated that various phenomena at the spinal cord level may be related to the referred pain pattern.[4,5] Specifically, the study demonstrated that pain stimulation of the receptive field of a nociceptor axon in a muscle resulted in the appearance of additional receptive fields in the same extremity. The sensitivity of the dorsal horn cell to noxious stimuli increased to include additional receptive fields. These studies implicate the spinal cord in referred pain pattern mechanisms.

Hong et al[5,6] found that when a needle penetrates the myofascial trigger point, referred pain is elicited 87.7% of the time, while palpation will elicit referred pain only 53.9% of the time.

REVIEW QUESTIONS

1. The presence of bradykinin, E-type prostaglandins, and 5-hydroxytrimptamine near the active loci can create sensitization effects contributing to the referred pain mechanism.
   True   False

2. Research has demonstrated that various phenomena at the spinal cord level are not related to the referred pain pattern.
   True   False

3. Palpation may elicit a referred pain pattern more frequently than needle insertion.
   True   False

REFERENCES

1. Selzer M, Spencer WA. Convergence of visceral and cutaneous afferent pathways in the lumbar spinal cord. *Brain Res.* 1969;14(2):331-348.

2. Selzer M, Spencer WA. Interactions between visceral and cutaneous afferents in the spinal cord: reciprocal primary afferent fiber depolarization. *Brain Res.* 1969;14(2)349-366.

3. Quintner JL, Cohen ML. Referred pain of peripheral nerve origin: an alternative to the "myofascial pain" construct. *Clin J Pain.* 1994;10:243-51.

4. Travell JG, Simons DG, Simons LS. *Myofascial Pain and Dysfunction: The Trigger Point Manual—Upper Half of Body.* Baltimore, Md: Williams & Wilkins; 1999.

5. Hong CZ, Simons DG. Pathophysiologic and electrophysiologic mechanisms of myofascial trigger points. *Arch Phys Med Rehabil.* 1998;79:863-72.

6. Hong CZ, Kuan TS, Chen JT, Chen SM. Referred pain elicited by palpation and by needling of myofascial trigger points: a comparison. *Arch Phys Med Rehabil.* 1997;78:957-60.

Chapter 7

CLASSIFICATION OF MYOFASCIAL TRIGGER POINTS

There are several ways to classify myofascial trigger points. Here we adopt the most frequently used in the literature and clinical practice.

ACTIVE TRIGGER POINT

An active myofascial trigger point produces pain without digital compression. It is very tender upon palpation; it produces a characteristic referred pain pattern for the muscle, either with ischemic compression or without; it impedes muscle flexibility; it produces muscle weakness; and it may elicit a local twitch response with compression or needle stimulation.

LATENT TRIGGER POINT

A latent myofascial trigger point is usually silent—without causing any spontaneous pain. However, it is tender upon palpation, it may produce a referred pain pattern only with the application of ischemic compression, it impedes muscle flexibility, it produces muscle weakness, and it may elicit a local twitch response with compression or needle stimulation. Latent myofascial trigger points may exist in the muscle for years following recovery from an injury. An active trigger point that was never treated or was improperly treated may become latent at a chronic stage. Latent trigger points may be reactivated and become active with microinjury/microtrauma or with a macrotrauma.

SATELLITE TRIGGER POINT

Satellite trigger points (Figure 7-1) may develop in the same muscle where the primary (main) trigger point is, in other muscles within the referred pain pattern of the primary trigger point, or in synergistic muscles. The satellite trigger point usually resolves once the main trigger point is resolved, without any additional intervention.

In their most recent text, Simons and Travell[1] make a distinction between central and attachment trigger points. They are defined below.

CENTRAL MYOFASCIAL TRIGGER POINT

A central myofascial trigger point is closely associated with dysfunctional endplates and is located near the center of muscle fibers.

ATTACHMENT TRIGGER POINT

An attachment trigger point (see Figure 7-1) is a trigger point at the musculotendinous junction and/or at the osseous attachment of the muscle that identifies the enthesopathy caused by unrelieved tension characteristic of the taut band that is produced by a central trigger point.

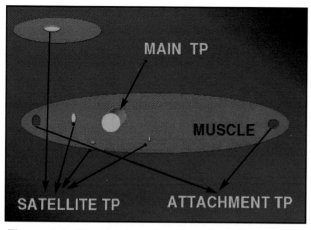

Figure 7-1. Classification of myofascial trigger points.

REFERENCE

1. Travell JG, Simons DG, Simons LS. *Myofascial Pain and Dysfunction: The Trigger Point Manual—Upper Half of Body.* Baltimore, Md: Williams & Wilkins; 1999.

REVIEW QUESTIONS

1. An active myofascial trigger point produces pain without digital compression.
   True   False

2. A latent myofascial trigger point is usually active and causes spontaneous pain.
   True   False

3. A latent myofascial trigger point has no effect on muscle flexibility and does not produce muscle tightness.
   True   False

4. An active trigger point that was never treated or was improperly treated may become latent at a chronic stage.
   True   False

5. Latent trigger points may be reactivated with microinjury/microtrauma or with macrotrauma.
   True   False

6. A myofascial trigger point that is closely associated with dysfunctional endplates and is located near the center of a muscle fiber is defined as a _____central_____ trigger point.

Chapter 8

BIOMECHANICS OF INJURY

An important component in the diagnosis of trigger point myofascial syndrome, especially when a decision must be made regarding the appropriate muscle to treat, is the biomechanics of the injury. One must consider the specific mechanism that may be responsible for the injury.

Using the referred pain pattern as the sole criterion to identify the muscle responsible for the dysfunction will produce inaccurate results because the referred pain patterns of several muscles overlap each other. Taking the patient's history and asking appropriate questions that will lead to identifying the possible mechanism of injury becomes very important. This process will help to piece together the diagnostic puzzle and, through deductive reasoning, arrive at correct conclusions regarding proper treatment.

Components that must be identified:

* Direction of external force applied (if the injury involved an external force).
* Relative position of the body during the injury.
* Specific movement that the body followed after application of the external force.
* Specific postural position that the patient usually assumes (if it is a postural dysfunction).
* Direction of habitual or repetitive movement (if it is a repetitive motion injury).
* Mechanics of the pelvis and spine in cases of skeletal asymmetries.
* Positional and functional anatomy of the feet in cases of faulty feet mechanics.

Careful inspection and observation may give hints regarding the biomechanics of injury; however, appropriate questions should be asked:

1. "Recalling the time of your injury, please describe or show me specifically how you fell."
2. "Recalling the exact way you move your wrist at work, please show me the specific movements involved."
3. "Recalling the exact way you sit while you watch television, please show me specifically how you sit?"

The least complicated cases to determine the biomechanics of injury are those that are the result of a high-velocity movement, such as sports injuries, sudden falls, and motor vehicle accidents. Patients injured through these mechanisms will easily recall the specific way they fell or were injured and the position their body assumed during that injury. However, injuries are not always the result of a high-velocity movement. Repetitive motion injuries, as well as injuries through stress positions, are very common. Manual laborers, musicians, and athletes engage in activities that require repetitive movement. Work stations that are not ergonomically correct will add further stress to joints and muscles.

The clinician must always ask the patient to specifically demonstrate the repetitive movement that may have caused the injury. Positions that put the muscles and joints under stress should also be considered. Postural and skeletal asymmetries, faulty posture, habitually biomechanically poor body positions, and stressed body positions over prolonged time may cause microtrauma and thus myofascial trigger point syndrome. This last category is the most challenging to obtain information from the patient regarding the biomechanics of injury because most of the time the patient is not conscious of certain positions or motions that caused the problem.

REVIEW QUESTIONS

1. The referred pain pattern is the sole criterion to identify the muscle responsible for the myofascial dysfunction.
    True   ~~False~~

2. Taking the patient's history and asking appropriate questions becomes very important and will lead to identifying the possible mechanism of injury.
    ~~True~~   False

3. Postural and skeletal asymmetries, faulty posture, habitually biomechanically poor body positions, and stress body positions over prolonged time may cause microtrauma and thus myofascial trigger point syndrome.
    ~~True~~   False

Chapter 9

MYOFASCIAL DIAGNOSIS

There are several steps that one must consider in the diagnosis of myofascial trigger point syndrome. Many times, the myofascial diagnosis may be secondary to the patient's problem. Physical and occupational therapists, as well as doctors of physical medicine and rehabilitation, frequently evaluate and treat patients who have been referred to them by a primary care physician, an orthopedist, a rheumatologist, a dentist, a podiatrist, and others. Frequently, the clinician who initially evaluated the patient may have established a nonmyofascial-type diagnosis and ignored a possible primary or secondary myofascial component to the dysfunction. Careful evaluation and assessment of the patient will frequently reveal that a cervical radiculopathy may have an associated sternocleidomastoid and scalenus myofascial trigger point syndrome; or a patient with pain in the heel and a primary diagnosis of inflammation due to a heel spur may have an associated tibialis posterior, soleus, and/or quadratus plantae myofascial trigger point syndrome. Therefore, it is important to further evaluate patients from a myofascial point of view and decide whether the myofascial component is a consequence of the primary diagnosis or a cause of it. In the latter scenario, the myofascial diagnosis should become the primary one.

DIAGNOSTIC TERMS

There are various expressions that can be used to describe a myofascial diagnosis. Some of them utilize the terms *myofascial dysfunction, myofascial syndrome, regional myofascial syndrome, myofascial pain syndrome,* and others.

The lack of consistency and use of vague expressions creates a problem in accurately defining terms and coming to an agreement about what each of these terms represents. In the authors' opinion, the most comprehensive term that has been used in the literature to describe the symptoms caused by a myofascial trigger point is *myofascial trigger point syndrome* (which we will adopt for this text). This term was introduced by David Simons, MD and we encourage clinicians and researchers to use this term in a consistent manner. Therefore, we use the name of the muscle that is myofascially involved followed by myofascial trigger point syndrome. Examples include iliopsoas myofascial trigger point syndrome, infraspinatus myofascial trigger point syndrome, etc.

RECOMMENDED CRITERIA TO IDENTIFY ACTIVE AND LATENT MYOFASCIAL TRIGGER POINTS

Studies by various researchers were reviewed regarding their validity and interrater reliability for accurate identification of myofascial trigger points.[1-7] Hsieh et al[4] reported poor interrater reliability in the identification by palpation of characteristics of myofascial trigger points; however, their interpretation of data and of the meaning of the Kappa values has been strongly challenged.[2] Gerwin et al[2,3] conducted an organized and detailed study and managed to obtain impressive Kappa values for the variables tested, indicating excellent reliability measures. Table 9-1 presents the variables tested and their results.

Table 9-1

INTERRATER RELIABILITY OF EXAMINATION OF TRIGGER POINTS[3,13]

Characteristic Examined	Kappa Value
Spot tenderness	0.84
Patient pain recognition	0.88
Palpable taut band	0.85
Referred pain pattern	0.69
Local twitch response	0.44
Mean score	0.74

Based on the variables studied by Gerwin et al[2,3,8,9] and suggestions made by Travell and Simons,[10-14] we adopt the following essential and confirmatory criteria for the accurate identification of latent and active myofascial trigger points.

ESSENTIAL CRITERIA

1. Palpable taut band: If the muscle is accessible, palpate for the taut band, which may include a tender nodule.
2. Exquisite spot tenderness of a nodule in a taut band: Palpating through a taut band, the clinician should identify the tender nodular area. Digital compression of the nodule may elicit a referred pain pattern (RPP).
3. Patient pain recognition: Digital ischemic compression on the tender nodule may reproduce the patient's pain symptom. Patients will usually identify that as "their usual pain." Patient pain recognition does not necessarily have to extend throughout the entire RPP, which is characteristic for the specific muscle. Eliciting the patient's pain recognition is a strong essential criterion and will discriminate an active trigger point from a latent one.
4. Painful range of motion at the end of range: It is a common characteristic of myofascial trigger points to restrict range of motion and produce pain at the end of the range. A painful muscle at the end of the range of movement should not be confused with the RPP or with the positive stretch sign (PSS).

CONFIRMATORY CRITERIA

1. Local twitch response (LTR): Eliciting a LTR may take place through snapping palpation across the taut band, especially across the fibers of the trigger point's active locus. LTR may be identified visually or through palpation.
2. Local twitch response via needle penetration: Eliciting an LTR may take place through needle pen-

etration at the area of the active locus. This area may include the immediate area of the trigger point as well as the immediate area around it.

3. Referred pain pattern: An RPP characteristic for the specific muscle may be elicited during digital compression on the area of the active locus.
4. Spontaneous electromyographic (EMG) activity: Presence of spontaneous EMG activity may occur when an EMG needle slowly approaches the area of active loci in the tender nodule of a taut band.

DIAGNOSTIC VALUE OF A REFERRED PAIN PATTERN

Identification of the RPP is an important and helpful confirmatory criterion to the diagnosis of a myofascial trigger point syndrome. In Travell and Simons' writings from the early 1980s,[15] great significance was placed on the RPP: "The patient's pattern of referred pain is usually the key to the diagnosis of a myofascial pain syndrome." In a recent algometry study[16] eliciting pressure over normal muscle tissue in subjects with myofascial trigger points, referred pain was elicited in 68% of patients with active trigger points and in 23.4% of patients with latent trigger points. In the same study, direct pressure over the trigger point elicited an RPP in all subjects with active myofascial trigger points but only in 46.8% of muscles with latent ones. When pressure was applied over any point of the taut band, an RPP was elicited again in all subjects with active myofascial trigger points but only in 36.2% with latent ones. Hong and Simons[17] concur that "referred pain is not a specific sign of a myofascial trigger point (MTrP), but it certainly occurs more often (and is much easier to elicit) in an active MTrP region than in a latent one or a normal muscle tissue."

As previously stated, it is the belief of the authors of this book that making a decision on what muscle to treat by looking only at the RPP may lead to a poor judgment. Often, patients present themselves with variable RPPs that belong to more than one muscle. At the same time, the RPP elicited by an active myofascial trigger point can be very different than the patient pain recognition. This complicates a diagnosis even further. Instead by placing primary importance on the essential trigger point criteria described above, with our assessment using the biomechanics of the injury we can arrive at the correct myofascial diagnosis with great precision.

MYOFASCIAL DIAGNOSIS

The following steps can be followed in myofascial diagnosis:

1. Take a history. Look for sudden onset from acute injury, trauma, overload stress; or gradual onset with chronic overload, microinjury, microtrauma, repetitive trauma. Objectively identify the patient's life problems from their point of view and understand their jobs, personal relationships, and other stressors of daily life.[18]
2. Establish biomechanics of injury from the history and questions-and-answers.
3. Palpate for a taut band: If the muscle is accessible, palpate for the taut band, which may include a tender nodule.
4. Identify tender nodules, usually within the taut band.
5. Identify patient pain recognition: Patient pain recognition does not necessarily have to extend throughout the entire RPP. The patient may identify the patient pain recognition sign in only a portion of the expected RPP. Differential diagnosis between an active trigger point and a latent one can be achieved with the presence of patient pain recognition.
6. Painful range of motion at the end of range. Pain at the attachments and/or the muscle belly may be present during end range of motion.
7. Identify possible local twitch response. Eliciting a LTR may take place through snapping palpation across the taut band. In cases of very high trigger point activity, mere compression of the trigger point may elicit an LTR.
8. Establish referred pain pattern: An RPP characteristic for the specific muscle may be elicited during digital compression on the area of the active locus. The RPP may be different from the patient pain recognition.
9. Identify possible weakness of the involved muscle. At times, application of manual muscle testing will demonstrate weakness of the myofascially involved muscle.
10. Correlate with other orthopedic/neurologic tests, including special tests and differential diagnostic tests.
11. Establish a diagnosis in myofascial terms.

REVIEW QUESTIONS

1. Digital ischemic compression on the tender nodule may reproduce the patient's pain symptom. This is called _pt. pain recognition_

2. A patient's pain recognition is one of the confirmatory criteria for the identification of a myofascial trigger point.
   True   False

3. A referred pain pattern is one of the essential criteria for the identification of a myofascial trigger point.
   True   False

4. Eliciting a patient's pain recognition is a very important criterion and will discriminate a _active_ trigger point from a _latent_ one.

5. Pain in the muscle at the end of the range of the movement is defined as positive stretch sign.
   True   False

6. Painful end range of motion is one of the essential criteria for the identification of a myofascial trigger point.
   True   False

7. Presence of spontaneous EMG activity when an EMG needle slowly approaches the area of active loci in the tender nodule of a taut band is one of the confirmatory criteria for the identification of a myofascial trigger point.
   True   False

REFERENCES

1. Fischer AA. Reliability of the pressure algometer as a measure of myofascial trigger point sensitivity. *Pain*. 1987;28:411-4.

2. Gerwin R, Shannon S. Interexaminer reliability and myofascial trigger points. *Arch Phys Med Rehabil*. 2000;81:1257-8.

3. Gerwin RD, Shannon S, Hong CZ, Hubbard D, Gevirtz R. Interrater reliability in myofascial trigger point examination. *Pain*. 1997;69:65-73.

4. Hsieh CY, Hong CZ, Adams AH, et al. Interexaminer reliability of the palpation of trigger points in the trunk and lower limb muscles. *Arch Phys Med Rehabil*. 2000;81:258-64.

5. Nice DA, Riddle DL, Lamb RL, Mayhew TP, Rucker K. Intertester reliability of judgments of the presence of trigger points in patients with low back pain. *Arch Phys Med Rehabil*. 1992;73:893-8.

6. Njoo KH, Van der Does E. The occurrence and inter-rater reliability of myofascial trigger points in the quadratus lumborum and gluteus medius: a prospective study in non-specific low back pain patients and controls in general practice. *Pain*. 1994;58:317-23.

7. Tunks E, McCain GA, Hart LE, et al. The reliability of examination for tenderness in patients with myofascial pain, chronic fibromyalgia and controls. *J Rheumatol*. 1995;22:944-52.

8. Gerwin RD. Neurobiology of the myofascial trigger point. *Baillieres Clin Rheumatol*. 1994;8:747-62.

9. Gerwin RD. Myofascial pain syndromes in the upper extremity. *J Hand Ther*. 1997;10:130-6.

10. Simons DG. Examining for myofascial trigger points. *Arch Phys Med Rehabil*. 1993;74:676-7.

11. Simons DG. The nature of myofascial trigger points. *Clin J Pain*. 1995;11:83-4.

12. Simons DG. Undiagnosed pain complaints: trigger points? *Clin J Pain*. 1997;13:82-3.

13. Travell JG, Simons DG, Simons LS. *Myofascial Pain and Dysfunction: The Trigger Point Manual—Upper Half of Body*. Baltimore, Md: Williams & Wilkins; 1999.

14. Wolfe F, Simons DG, Fricton J, et al. The fibromyalgia and myofascial pain syndromes: a preliminary study of tender points and trigger points in persons with fibromyalgia, myofascial pain syndrome and no disease. *J Rheumatol*. 1992;19:944-51.

15. Travell JG, Simons DG. *Myofascial Pain and Dysfunction: The Trigger Point Manual*. Vol 1. Baltimore, Md: Williams & Wilkins; 1983.

16. Hong CZ, Chen YN, Twehous D, Hong D. Pressure threshold for referred pain by compression on the trigger point and adjacent areas. *J Musculoskel Pain*. 1996;61-79.

17. Hong CZ, Simons DG. Pathophysiologic and electrophysiologic mechanisms of myofascial trigger points. *Arch Phys Med Rehabil*. 1998;79:863-72.

18. Travell J. *Advances in Pain Research and Therapy: Chronic Myofascial Pain Syndromes Mysteries of the History*. New York: Raven Press Ltd; 1990;17:129-137.

Chapter 10

MYOFASCIAL TREATMENT

After myofascial diagnosis has been established, the following treatment sequence can be applied.

1. Modalities to the affected muscle. The application of heat and other modalities (hot packs, cold packs, ultrasound, etc) to the involved muscle will help increase blood circulation in the area and promote relaxation. Duration and method of application varies depending on the modality selected. The clinician must consider all applicable contraindications before the application of any modality. Some of the possible modalities are:

   * Hot packs to promote a general increase in blood circulation and a feeling of relaxation. Apply for 15 to 20 minutes over the involved muscle.

   * Ultrasound as a heating modality will transmit vibrational energy up to approximately 5 cm, generating heat within the tissue. The exact mechanism on how ultrasound may benefit in the treatment of myofascial trigger points must be further researched. Pulsed ultrasound may be used over a myofascial trigger point. Application of continuous ultrasound will require continuous movement of the sonic head during its application. There are no studies available to indicate the effectiveness of one method versus the other on myofascial trigger points.

   * Phonophoresis and iontophoresis to deliver drugs, such as hydrocortisone, lidocaine, and others. The low level of penetration, up to 1 cm under the skin, makes it difficult for the drug to reach the submuscular tissue.

   * Electrical stimulation in various forms has been used in the treatment of myofascial trigger points.

The authors of this book utilize an alternating (not continuous) current and increase the intensity to the point in which quick but gentle muscular contractions are produced. The application of this kind of electrical stimulation may have a similar effect as eliciting an LTR during dry needling. At the same time, the muscle seems to fatigue and a further degree of relaxation is achieved. Electrical stimulation may also be applied with the use of a probe over the trigger point.

   * Low-level laser therapy (LLLT) applied over the area of a trigger point with three 15-second applications has been found to be very effective in normalizing skin resistance, which is an indication of myofascial trigger point normalization.[1] LLLT is usually applied with helium-neon 632.8 nm (nanometers) visible red or infrared 820 to 830 nm continuous wave and 904 nm pulsed emission.[2] Recent studies[1-3] indicate a decrease in muscle rigidity, increase of mobility, and a decrease in pain[4-6] in muscles with myofascial trigger points. LLLT improves local microcirculation, increases oxygen supply to hypoxic cells in the trigger point areas, and at the same time can help remove collected waste products. According to Tam,[6] the semiconductor or laser diode (GaAs, 904 nm) is the most appropriate choice in pain reduction therapy. A low-power density laser acts on the prostaglandin (PG) synthesis, increasing the change of PGG2 and PGH2 into PG12 (also called prostacyclin or epoprostenol). The latter is the main product of the arachidonic acid into the endothelial cells and into the smooth muscular cells of vessel walls, which have a vasodilating and

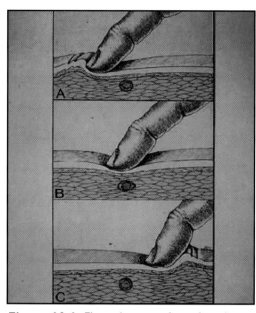

Figure 10-1. Flat palpation of myofascial trigger points using the thumb or fingers (reprinted with permission from Travell JG, Simons DG, Simons LS. *Myofascial Pain and Dysfunction The Trigger Point Manual—Upper Half of Body.* Baltimore, Md: Williams & Wilkins; 1999).

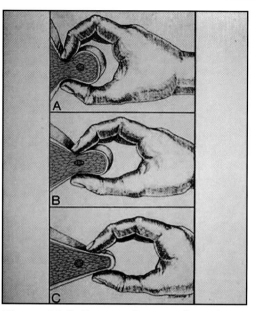

Figure 10-2. Pincer palpation of myofascial trigger points (reprinted with permission from Travell JG, Simons DG, Simons LS. *Myofascial Pain and Dysfunction The Trigger Point Manual—Upper Half of Body.* Baltimore, Md: Williams & Wilkins; 1999).

anti-inflammatory action. Simunovic[3,7] reports that pain diminished in 70% of individuals with acute pain and in 60% of individuals with chronic pain after the application of LLLT. (An important point must be noted: no modality may replace the manual therapeutic intervention provided by the clinician.)

2. Trigger point therapy can be applied in various forms. These include:

* Progressive pressure technique: This manual therapy technique requires the use of hands or fingers and can be applied in the form of flat palpation (Figure 10-1) or pincer palpation (Figure 10-2). The clinician may use the thumbs or the fingers, the knuckles, the elbows, or a combination of all to apply pressure. Rather than applying a fast ischemic compression on the tissue that will create excessive pain and muscle guarding, we utilize a more gentle technique called *progressive pressure technique*. The technique is performed as follows: Use the thumbs or four fingers of one or both hands and apply steady pressure, moving inward toward the center. Once tissue resistance is felt, stop and wait until resistance dissipates. At this point, the clinician may feel a slow release or a "melting away" sensation of the tissue under the treating fingers. The clinician should then proceed with further steady pressure, moving again inward

toward the center. Once new tissue resistance appears, the clinician should stop and wait with steady force against the tissue, then repeat this cycle several times. At the end, either further relaxation of the tissue will be felt or no new gains will be achieved. The muscle should be placed in a relaxed position but not a very shortened one. Pressure application varies in quantity and may start from a few ounces up to a couple of pounds. The clinician should always be guided by the patient's pain tolerance, and constant feedback should be provided by the patient.

Several other techniques set a time limitation to the application of the digital compression. The authors do not believe that such a limitation is necessary, provided that the clinician treats within reason. We usually apply this progressive pressure technique for at least 30 seconds to up to 2 minutes at a time. The treatment will finally release the contractured sarcomeres of the contraction knots in the myofascial trigger point area.[8-11] Travell calls a similar technique "ischemic compression" because upon release, the skin is at first blanched and then shows reactive hyperemia.[11,12] The patient should breathe deeply and slowly while the clinician progressively increases the pressure. Deep relaxation is very important for effectiveness of the technique.

Some clinicians may use different types of trigger point treatment devices that allow them to apply the trigger point techniques without discomfort to their fingers and hands.

* Postisometric relaxation, reciprocal inhibition, contract-relax technique, muscle energy technique, strain-counterstrain technique, massage and myofascial release techniques may all affect myofascial trigger points in various ways. This text, however, emphasizes the progressive pressure technique as the treatment of choice.

* Trigger point dry needling is a very effective approach that uses a fine flexible needle (usually an acupuncture needle) to elicit LTRs from the trigger point and finally inactivate it.

* Trigger point injections using a nonmyotoxic local anesthetic can be useful. Lidocaine 0.5%[13] or a procaine injection[11,12,14] has been recommended by various researchers; however, eliciting an LTR during the procedure is of utmost importance.[13] Since the origin of myofascial trigger points lies on the premise of dysfunctional endplates, sensible use of botulinum toxin A has been found to be effective in inactivating trigger points.[15-19]

3. For effective trigger point therapy, it must always be followed by myofascial stretching (MFS) exercises. Travell and Simons state "the key to treating trigger points is to lengthen the muscle fibers that are shortened by the trigger point mechanism."[10] To efficiently deliver power to a movement, a muscle is placed in a gentle stretch before performing a shortening contraction. Before an activity is performed, a muscle must be able to properly stretch and lengthen without causing injury to other structures in the musculoskeletal system. An injured muscle loses this property. Therefore, after the clinician helps the muscle relax by inactivating the trigger point via progressive pressure technique, he or she must stretch the muscle to maintain the degree of relaxation and bring the muscle to an ergonomically correct state. In other words, inactivation of the myofascial trigger points should be followed by lengthening the overshortened sarcomeres. An increase in the range of motion immediately following passive stretch has been identified in the literature and can be explained by the viscoelastic behavior of muscle and short-term changes in muscle extensibility.[20,21] Passive stretch that exceeds 30 seconds can be sufficient to obtain increased mobility.[22]

De Deyne, in a recent study,[23] identified that mobility gained through rehabilitation-type stretching produces a permanent adaptive response since the mobility is maintained. Apparently, through the process of myofibrilogenesis, a stretched muscle fiber ultimately leads to a longer muscle fiber with more sarcomeres in series.[24] The stretching technique appropriate for myofascially involved muscles must take into account the pathologic overshortening of the involved muscle fibers. To make a clear distinction about the specific way this stretching should be performed, we call it *myofascial stretching*. When there is an active trigger point in a muscle, only a portion of specific muscle fibers is involved. If someone performs a general, relatively fast stretch in this muscle, all healthy, noninvolved fibers will stretch. At the same time, the sarcomeres above and below the trigger point locus will overstretch to accommodate the change in muscle length, while the shortened trigger point area will develop an increase in tension during this fast stretch. On the contrary, myofascial stretch is very specific in isolating the muscle and very slow in rate to actually affect these myofascially involved fibers.

Proper myofascial stretching requires deep relaxation with proper concentration and breathing. This will inhibit the "gamma spindle" response. The gamma spindle system is a servo-mechanism (biofeedback system) within a muscle that causes the muscle to shorten when rapidly stretched.[24] The response of the gamma spindle is rate dependent (ie, only rapid lengthening causes the muscle to contract, whereas a slow rate of deformation will not elicit a response). The muscle must be allowed to "relax out" rather than "push through." This is a subtle difference that requires concentration on what is occurring in the patient's body.

MFS is different than regular stretching in the sense that it is very specific for the muscle under treatment and requires a narrow therapeutic range.[25] Overstretching during the application of MFS should be avoided and absolute relaxation must be achieved.

Ingber[25] suggests the following sequence for the application of MFS:

* Place the muscle to be stretched at the position where tension is sensed in the target muscle, at the end range of motion.

* While exhaling, allow the muscle to relax so that it stretches to an increased length.

* Hold the newly gained position while inhaling.

* Gain further length with each succeeding exhalation for 20 to 45 seconds, moving at the rate of 3 to 4 mm/sec, allowing the muscle to "relax out" rather than "push through."[25]

To ensure the MFS is performed correctly, the clinician must be very clear and thorough when instructing the patient.

Caution: During the application of MFS, eliciting a positive stretch sign (PSS) is an indication that the clinician or patient is pushing through the stretch more than necessary. In that case, the clinician should either decrease the amount of MFS or return the muscle to a relaxed position and perform additional trigger point therapy before additional MFS is performed. MFS will be given to the patient as a home exercise program and should be repeated four to six times daily with two repetitions each time.

Vapocoolant spray may be used in a spray and stretch technique to inactivate acute myofascial trigger points.[11,26] Ethyl chloride[27,28] or fluorimethane[10,29] can be effectively used. There are, however, environmental concerns regarding both products and an informed decision about their use must be made. The clinician should carefully read the manufacturer's product information and guidelines. The recommended treatment method when using vapocoolant spray follows (Figure 10-3):

* Have the patient sit in a relaxed position and position the muscle until slight tension is felt.
* Hold the spray bottle 8 to 12 inches above the skin and spray three sweeps from above the trigger point area but into the RPP zone, continue through the trigger point area, then below the trigger point area but into the RPP zone.
* After three sweeps have been applied, gently stroke the skin with your palm into the same direction as the spraying.
* Apply gentle stretch, allowing the muscle to elongate.
* Repeat the same cycle up to three consecutive times, always being aware that if a PSS develops, the technique must immediately stop. Always remember that pain or tension felt directly from the muscle that has been stretched does not qualify as a PSS.

4. Post-treatment modalities. If the skin is sore or if post-injection soreness persists, apply cold packs to decrease sensitivity in the area.

5. Muscle strengthening exercise sequence. Muscle strengthening exercises are important and should be applied as part of the myofascial treatment. Usually, the clinician will notice an increase in muscle strength right after the application of MFS.[25,30,31] However, a systematic muscle strengthening program should be applied as part of the treatment. The authors of this book initiate muscle strengthening exercises after the patient has achieved 70% combined range of motion of the involved muscle and joint.[32,33] The following sequence of muscle strengthening exercises is recommended:

* Isometric strengthening in various ranges of motion

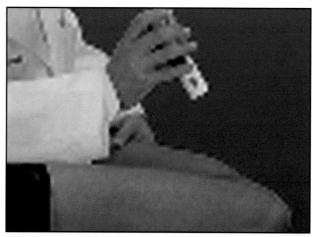

Figure 10-3. Application of the spray and stretch technique enables the clinician to achieve an increased muscle length, avoiding local muscle discomfort and muscle guarding (video screen capture).

* Low-resistance isotonic strengthening exercises
* Moderate resistance isotonic strengthening
* Isokinetic strengthening, starting with concentric-concentric and progressing to concentric-eccentric contractions
* Maximum resistance isotonic exercise
* Throughout this strengthening program, safe closed kinetic chain exercises should be performed both as clinic training and as a home exercise program

6. Proprioceptive training. Microtrauma and myofascial trigger points in a muscle create uncoordinated muscle function.[34-37] Contraction rate in the muscle increases and, therefore, the time it takes for a muscle to recruit the maximum number of motor units required for a specific contraction slows down. To prevent injury—especially microinjury—fast reflex muscle contraction is required to protect the involved joints.[35,36,38] During proprioceptive training, a clinician or an instrument introduces unexpected external forces of random frequency, magnitude, and direction to different parts of the patient's body, facilitating various receptors. The goal is to increase proprioceptive flow and facilitate the proprioceptive system, especially those pathways responsible for equilibrium, posture, and muscle control.[36] Various devices, such as trampolines, balance and rocker boards, balance shoes, and others have been used to facilitate the receptors (Figures 10-4 and 10-5).

7. Home exercise program. Patients must be instructed in self-stretching exercises to be performed between treatments. It is very important that patients understand how to correctly perform a MFS. The patient

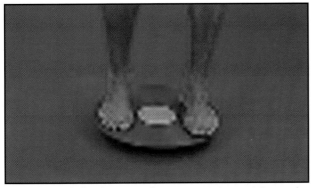

Figure 10-4. Application of proprioceptive training techniques (video screen capture).

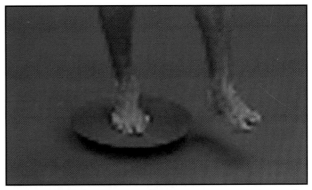

Figure 10-5. Application of proprioceptive training techniques (video screen capture).

can apply the MFS four to six times daily. Recent research[26] demonstrated that a home exercise program that consisted of ischemic pressure and sustained stretching was found to be effective in reducing sensitivity of myofascial trigger points and decreasing pain intensity in individuals with neck and upper back pain. When the clinician introduces the muscle strengthening exercise sequence or proprioceptive training, appropriate home exercises should be given to the patient.

REVIEW QUESTIONS

1. Heating modalities may help to increase blood circulation at the trigger point area and promote overall relaxation.
   True   False

2. According to the progressive pressure technique, 15 to 20 pounds of force must be applied on the trigger point.
   True   False

3. Application of the trigger point therapy should take place with the muscle in its maximum shortened position.
   True   False

4. Application of the trigger point therapy should take place with the muscle in its maximum lengthened position.
   True   False

5. Myofascial stretch is very specific in isolating the muscle and very slow in rate to actually affect the myofascially involved fibers.
   True   False

6. During the myofascial stretch, the clinician hopes to activate the muscle spindle.
   True   False

7. Myofascial stretching is different than regular stretching in that it is very specific for the muscle under treatment and requires a narrow therapeutic range.
   True   False

8. The goal of proprioceptive training is to increase proprioceptive flow and facilitate the proprioceptive system, especially those pathways responsible for equilibrium, posture, and muscle control.
   True   False

9. A 25-year-old dancer presents with left heel pain. After careful evaluation and biomechanical analysis, it becomes obvious that the patient has active myofascial trigger points in the left tibialis posterior muscle. What is likely the most proper intervention?
   A. Treat with modalities and apply trigger point therapy and myofascial stretching exercises to the left tibialis posterior. Provide a regular home exercise program.
   B. Treat with modalities and apply myofascial stretching exercises to the left tibialis posterior.

No need for trigger point therapy because the patient is very active as a dancer and the trigger point will resolve by itself. Provide a regular home exercise program.

C. Treat with modalities and apply trigger point therapy to the left tibialis posterior. No need for myofascial stretching exercises because the patient stretches frequently as a dancer. Provide a regular home exercise program.

D. Treat with modalities and apply trigger point therapy and myofascial stretching exercises to the left tibialis posterior.

10. A patient has an immobilized shoulder due to an open rotator cuff repair. He has active trigger points in the subscapularis muscle and abduction is limited to 85 degrees. According to the authors' philosophy and method of treatment, what is likely the most appropriate intervention?

A. Patient should receive modalities, trigger point therapy, and myofascial stretching exercises for the subscapularis muscle and isokinetic strengthening for the subscapularis.

B. The patient should receive modalities, trigger point therapy, and myofascial stretching exercises for the subscapularis muscle. A muscle strengthening exercise program for the subscapularis should be initiated as soon as the patient reaches 100 degrees of abduction. Gentle muscle strengthening that addresses other muscles can be immediately initiated.

C. The patient should receive modalities, trigger point therapy, and myofascial stretching exercises for the subscapularis muscle. A muscle strengthening exercise program for the subscapularis should be initiated as soon as the patient reaches 125 degrees of abduction. Gentle muscle strengthening that addresses other muscles can be immediately initiated.

D. The patient should receive modalities, trigger point therapy, and myofascial stretching exercises for the subscapularis muscle. A muscle strengthening exercise program for the subscapularis should be initiated as soon as the patient reaches 155 degrees of abduction. Gentle muscle strengthening that addresses other muscles can be immediately initiated.

REFERENCES

1. Snyder-Mackler L, Bork C, Bourbon B, Trumbore D. Effect of helium-neon laser on musculoskeletal trigger points. *Phys Ther.* 1986;66:1087-90.

2. Simunovic Z. Low level laser therapy with trigger points technique: a clinical study on 243 patients. *J Clin Laser Med Surg.* 1996;14:163-7.

3. Simunovic Z, Trobonjaca T, Trobonjaca Z. Treatment of medial and lateral epicondylitis—tennis and golfer's elbow—with low level laser therapy: a multicenter double blind, placebo-controlled clinical study on 324 patients. *J Clin Laser Med Surg.* 1998;16:145-51.

4. Ceccherelli F, Altafini L, Lo Castro G, Avila A, Ambrosio F, Giron GP. Diode laser in cervical myofascial pain: a double-blind study versus placebo. *Clin J Pain.* 1989;5:301-4.

5. Sieron A, Adamek M, Cieslar G, Zmudzinski J. Personal experience in clinical use of low power laser therapy. *Przegl Lek.* 1995;52:13-5.

6. Tam G. Low power laser therapy and analgesic action. *J Clin Laser Med Surg.* 1999;17:29-33.

7. Simunovic Z. Low level laser therapy with trigger points technique: a clinical study on 243 patients. *J Clin Laser Med Surg.* 1996;14:163-7.

8. Simons DG. Myofascial pain syndromes. *Arch Phys Med Rehabil.* 1984;65:561.

9. Travell JG, Simons DG. *Myofascial Pain and Dysfunction: The Trigger Point Manual—The Lower Extremities.* Media, Pa: Williams & Wilkins; 1983.

10. Travell JG, Simons DG, Simons LS. *Myofascial Pain and Dysfunction: The Trigger Point Manual—Upper Half of Body.* Baltimore, Md: Williams & Wilkins; 1999.

11. Travell JG, Simons DG. *Myofascial Pain and Dysfunction: The Trigger Point Manual.* Vol 1. Baltimore, Md: Williams & Wilkins; 1983.

12. Simons DG, Travell JG. Myofascial origins of low back pain. 1. Principles of diagnosis and treatment. *Postgrad Med.* 1983;73:66, 68-70, 73 passim.

13. Hong CZ. Lidocaine injection versus dry needling to myofascial trigger point. The importance of the local twitch response. *Am J Phys Med Rehabil.* 1994;73:256-63.

14. Travell JG, Rinzler S, Herman M. Pain and disability of the shoulder and arm: treatment by intramuscular infiltration with procaine hydrochloride. *JAMA.* 1942;120:417-422.

15. Acquadro MA, Borodic GE. Treatment of myofascial pain with botulinum A toxin. *Anesthesiology.* 1994;80:705-6.

16. Cheshire WP, Abashian SW, Mann JD. Botulinum toxin in the treatment of myofascial pain syndrome. *Pain.* 1994;59:65-9.

17. Diaz JH, Gould HJ III. Management of post-thoracotomy pseudoangina and myofascial pain with botulinum toxin. *Anesthesiology.* 1999;91:877-9.

18. Gerwin RD. Neurobiology of the myofascial trigger point. *Baillieres Clin Rheumatol.* 1994;8:747-62.

19. Porta M. A comparative trial of botulinum toxin type A and methylprednisolone for the treatment of myofascial pain syndrome and pain from chronic muscle spasm. *Pain.* 2000;85:101-5.

20. Best TM. Soft-tissue injuries and muscle tears. *Clin Sports Med.* 1997;16:419-34.

21. Best TM, McElhaney J, Garrett WE, Myers BS. Characterization of the passive responses of live skeletal muscle using the quasi-linear theory of viscoelasticity. *J Biomech.* 1994;27:413-9.

22. Bandy WD, Irion JM. The effect of time on static stretch on the flexibility of the hamstring muscles. *Phys Ther.* 1994;74:845-52.

23. De Deyne PG. Application of passive stretch and its implications for muscle fibers. *Phys Ther.* 2001;81:819-827.

24. Kandel E, Schartz J, Jessell TM. *Principles of Neural Science.* 4th ed. New York: McGraw-Hill; 2000.

25. Ingber R. *Myofascial Pain in Lumbar Dysfunction.* Philadelphia, Pa: Hanley & Belfus Inc; 1999.

26. Hanten WP, Olson SL, Butts NL, Nowicki AL. Effectiveness of a home program of ischemic pressure followed by sustained stretch for treatment of myofascial trigger points. *Phys Ther.* 2000;80:997-1003.

27. Gunn C. *The Gunn Approach to the Treatment of Chronic Pain—Intramuscular Stimulation for Myofascial Pain of Radiculopathic Origin.* London: Churchill Livingstone; 1996.

28. Marcus N, Kraus H, Rachlin E. Comments on KH Njoo and E. Van der Does, *Pain,* 58 (1994) 317-323. *Pain.* 1995;61:159.

29. Simons DG, Travell JG, Simons LS. Protecting the ozone layer. *Arch Phys Med Rehabil.* 1990;71:64.

30. Ingber RS. Shoulder impingement in tennis/racquetball players treated with subscapularis myofascial treatments. *Arch Phys Med Rehabil.* 2000;81:679-82.

31. Wilson GJ, Elliott BC, Wood GA. Stretch shorten cycle performance enhancement through flexibility training. *Med Sci Sports Exerc.* 1992;24:116-23.

32. Kostopoulos D, Rizopoulos K. Trigger point and myofascial therapy. *Advance for Physical Therapists.* 1998:25-28.

33. Kostopoulos D, Rizopoulos K, Brown A. Shin splint pain: the runner's nemesis. *Advance for Physical Therapists.* 1999:33-34.

34. Freeman M, Dean M, Hanham I. The etiology and prevention of functional instability of the foot. *J Bone Joint Surg Br.* 1965;678.

35. Janda V. Muscle strength in relation to muscle length, pain and muscle imbalance. *International Perspectives in Physical Therapy.* New York: Churchill Livingstone; 1993;8:83-91.

36. Janda V, Va'Vrota M. Sensory motor stimulation. In: Liebenson C. *Rehabilitation of the Spine.* Baltimore, Md: Williams & Wilkins; 1996:319-328.

37. Kurtz A. Chronic sprained ankle. *Am J Surg.* 1939;158.

38. Twomey L, Janda V. *Physical Therapy of the Low Back: Muscles and Motor Control in Low Back Pain: Assessment and Management.* New York: Churchill Livingstone; 253-278; 2000.

Chapter 11

PERPETUATING FACTORS IN MYOFASCIAL TRIGGER POINTS

It is a very common phenomenon when treating patients with a chronic or unresolved myofascial trigger point syndrome to see that other exogenous factors may have a negative effect on the condition. Usually, these patients do well immediately following the treatment, but a couple of days later they regress to the initial state. The reason for that regression is an uncontrolled—and possibly unknown to the patient and to the clinician—factor that perpetuates the dysfunction. These are called perpetuating factors and can be related to abnormal body positions, postural positions, skeletal asymmetries, as well as activities that increase mechanical stresses causing reactivation of myofascial trigger points.

Examples of such conditions include:

* An asymmetry such as a leg length discrepancy that exceeds 0.5 to 1 cm. Such a discrepancy will cause muscular asymmetries that will extend from the lower extremity to the sacroiliac joint, the pelvis, and further to the spine, producing abnormal stresses.
* Muscle imbalances can become stressors that will activate myofascial trigger points. For example, tightness on the right biceps femoris (long head) will produce abnormal tension on the ipsilateral sacrotuberus ligament. This is connected to the fascia of the contralateral gluteus maximus, which has a direct connection to the thoracolumbar fascia, the furthest part of the fascia of the latissimus dorsi. Abnormal stresses, tension, and overload may create myofascial trigger points in any of the muscles mentioned here. It becomes obvious how important it is to thoroughly evaluate the patient. Only then can the clinician manage to identify such perpetuating factors and correct them.
* A classic example of an iatrogenic perpetuating factor is to provide the patient with a cane of improper length. Continuous use of a cane that is either too tall or too short will cause asymmetries and will apply abnormal stresses to the muscles of the upper body.

Nutritional factors may play a role in the perpetuation of a myofascial trigger point syndrome. It is recommended that patients with a chronic myofascial trigger point syndrome take vitamins B_1, B_6, B_{12}, folic acid, and vitamin C.

Metabolic and endocrine inadequacies, as well as psychological and behavioral issues, may act as perpetuating factors in a myofascial trigger point syndrome. The clinician should be able to identify such factors and make appropriate referrals if the issue is outside the scope of his or her practice.

REVIEW QUESTIONS

1. Perpetuating factors are factors that are uncontrolled and possibly unknown to the clinician and patient that prolong a patient's myofascial dysfunction.
   True   False

2. Perpetuating factors can be related to abnormal body positions, postural positions, and skeletal asymmetries, as well as activities that increase mechanical stresses causing reactivation of myofascial trigger points.
   True   False

3. Nutritional factors play no role in the perpetuation of a myofascial trigger point syndrome.
   True   False

4. A patient presents with pain in the right sacroiliac and gluteal region. Myofascial evaluation reveals presence of an active myofascial trigger point on the gluteus medius muscle. Further evaluation reveals a Morton's foot condition (second metatarsal longer and lower than the first, causing foot pronation, tibial rotation, femoral adduction, and internal rotation during ambulation). What is the recommended treatment plan?
   A. Treat the gluteus medius muscle myofascially and stretch the heel to correct the foot condition.
   B. Consider Morton's foot as a perpetuating factor. Resolve Morton's foot with the proper orthotic device and treat the gluteus medius muscle myofascially.
   C. Consider Morton's foot as a perpetuating factor. Resolve Morton's foot with the proper orthotic device. No treatment is necessary for the gluteus medius because the muscle has an active trigger point and will resolve by itself.
   D. Treat the gluteus medius muscle myofascially and stretch the second metatarsal to correct the foot condition.

Chapter 12

TRIGGER POINT DRY NEEDLING

Trigger point dry needling technique involves insertion and repetitive manipulation of a fine and flexible needle in the trigger point of a muscle to produce a local twitch response, resulting in muscle relaxation.

Travell and Simons,[1] in *Myofascial Pain and Dysfunction: The Trigger Point Manual*, state that there are several ways to treat trigger points, including spray and stretch, ischemic compression, injection with saline or local anesthetic, and dry needling. Dry needling requires the greatest precision and the most repetition. There are several studies providing evidence that dry needling is more effective than other techniques, including local anesthetics.[2,3]

In 1979, Lewit,[4,5] in his study published in *Pain*, demonstrated the effectiveness of dry needling. Frost et al[6-10] demonstrated that injection of normal saline into the trigger point was more effective than injecting a local anesthetic. They proposed that it was not the injectable material that they used, but the needling procedure itself that produced such results. Inserting the needle at the site caused a stimulation of the reflex arc. Because the afferent pathway was the muscle, the muscle relaxed.[6,8] Therefore, relaxation of the muscle was obtained through the spinal reflex arc.

In a clinical trial of 58 patients with myofascial trigger points on the upper trapezius muscle, application of trigger point dry needling technique was found to be equally effective as injection with 0.5% lidocaine in reducing pain intensity, muscle pressure sensitivity on pressure algometry, and cervical range of motion.[2] Trigger point dry needling produced a higher incidence of local post-treatment soreness. Hong and others, however, emphasized the importance of eliciting a local twitch response (LTR) during the application of any needling technique.[2,11-14]

The mechanism of dry needling action that seems to provide muscle relaxation and pain relief, according to Fischer, is that dry needling mechanically breaks up the nodularity of the tissue.[15-17] Gunn supports that there is a histamine release that causes local irritation and relaxation of the muscle.[18] In Ingber's opinion, the mechanism of action is one of a decrease in the stiffness of the muscle we are treating through an electrical event.[19] Decrease of stiffness increases the flexibility of the muscle that is maintained through the myofascial stretching exercises.[20-22]

The advantage of dry needling techniques over other techniques is that we can establish a painless full range of motion at the time of treatment (immediate response). It also improves a kinesthetic sense, because we can immediately teach the patient full painless range of motion, which is the ultimate aim of myofascial treatment. Other advantages of dry needling include absence of allergic reactions, decreased chance of hematomas, and treatment of deep muscles close to neurovascular bundles. The disadvantage is that the technique is painful and may produce post-treatment soreness.

Trigger point dry needling is an invasive procedure and should be applied only by those clinicians whose state licenses permit such practice. Dry needling must not be confused with acupuncture.

REVIEW QUESTIONS

1. Trigger point dry needling technique involves insertion and repetitive manipulation of a fine and flexible needle into the trigger point area of a muscle.
   True   False

2. A local twitch response during a dry needling session is an unwanted event and results in harming the muscle.
   True   False

3. The mechanism of dry needling action that seems to provide muscle relaxation and pain relief, according to Fischer, is that dry needling mechanically breaks up the nodularity of the tissue.
   True   False

4. Ingber supports that there is a histamine release that causes local irritation and relaxation of the muscle.
   True   False

5. A disadvantage of dry needling is that it is painful and may produce post-treatment soreness.
   True   False

6. Trigger point dry needling is an invasive procedure and should be applied only by those clinicians whose state licenses permit such practice.
   True   False

REFERENCES

1. Travell JG, Simons DG. *Myofascial Pain and Dysfunction: The Trigger Point Manual.* Vol 1. Baltimore, Md: Williams & Wilkins; 1983.

2. Hong CZ. Lidocaine injection versus dry needling to myofascial trigger point. The importance of the local twitch response. *Am J Phys Med Rehabil.* 1994;73:256-63.

3. Hong CZ, Kuan TS, Chen JT, Chen SM. Referred pain elicited by palpation and by needling of myofascial trigger points: a comparison. *Arch Phys Med Rehabil.* 1997;78:957-60.

4. Lewit K. The needle effect in the relief of myofascial pain. *Pain.* 1979;6:83-90.

5. Lewit K. *Manipulative Therapy in Rehabilitation of the Locomotor System.* Oxford, England: Butterworth-Heinemann; 1999.

6. Frost A. Diclofenac versus lidocaine as injection therapy in myofascial pain. *Scand J Rheumatol.* 1986;15:153-6.

7. Frost A. Diclofenac compared with lidocaine in the treatment of myofascial pain by injections. *Ugeskr Laeger.* 1986;148:1077-8.

8. Frost FA, Jessen B, Siggaard-Andersen J. A controlled double-blind comparison of mepivacaine injection versus saline injection for myofascial pain. *Lancet.* 1980;1:499-500.

9. Frost FA, Jessen B, Siggaard-Andersen J. Myofascial pain treated with injections. A controlled double-blind trial. *Ugeskr Laeger.* 1980;142:1754-7.

10. Frost FA, Toft B, Aaboe T. Isotonic saline and methylprednisolone acetate in blockade treatment of myofascial pain. A clinical controlled study. *Ugeskr Laeger.* 1984;146:652-4.

11. Hong CZ, Hsueh TC. Difference in pain relief after trigger point injections in myofascial pain patients with and without fibromyalgia. *Arch Phys Med Rehabil.* 1996;77:1161-6.

12. Hong CZ, Simons DG. Pathophysiologic and electrophysiologic mechanisms of myofascial trigger points. *Arch Phys Med Rehabil.* 1998;79:863-72.

13. Simons DG. The nature of myofascial trigger points. *Clin J Pain.* 1995;11:83-4.

14. Simons D, Hong C, Simons LS. Nature of myofascial trigger points, active loci. *Journal of Musculoskeletal Pain.* 1995;3(1Suppl):62.

15. Fischer AA. Reliability of the pressure algometer as a measure of myofascial trigger point sensitivity. *Pain.* 1987;28:411-4.

16. Fischer AA. Documentation of myofascial trigger points. *Arch Phys Med Rehabil.* 1988;69:286-91.

17. Kraus H, Fischer AA. Diagnosis and treatment of myofascial pain. *Mt Sinai J Med.* 1991;58:235-9.

18. Gunn C. *The Gunn Approach to the Treatment of Chronic Pain—Intramuscular Stimulation for Myofascial Pain of Radiculopathic Origin.* London: Churchill Livingstone; 1996.

19. Ingber R. Personal communication; 1991.

20. Ingber RS. Iliopsoas myofascial dysfunction: a treatable cause of "failed" low back syndrome. *Arch Phys Med Rehabil.* 1989;70:382-6.

21. Ingber RS. Shoulder impingement in tennis/racquetball players treated with subscapularis myofascial treatments. *Arch Phys Med Rehabil.* 2000;81:679-82.

22. Ingber R. *Myofascial Pain in Lumbar Dysfunction.* Philadelphia, Pa: Hanley & Belfus Inc; 1999.

Chapter 13

TRIGGER POINT AND MYOFASCIAL THERAPY CONTRAINDICATIONS

When patients suffer from one or more of the following conditions, trigger point and myofascial therapy may be contraindicated:

* Malignancy: When a mass of cancer cells may invade surrounding tissues or spread to distant areas of the body. In general, manual therapy may be contraindicated depending on the type and area of the tumor.

* Open wounds in the area of application of trigger point therapy. Tissue may become more irritated with the application of trigger point therapy and myofascial stretching exercises.

* Severe arteriosclerosis: Commonly shows its effects first in the legs and feet. The arteries may become narrowed and blood flow decreases, progressing in some cases to total closure (occlusion) of the vessel. The vessel walls become less elastic and cannot dilate to allow greater blood flow when needed. Excessive compression and stretching may cause blood clot formation.

* Aneurysm: Resembles a sack of blood attached to one side of a blood vessel by a narrow neck. All types of manual therapy are contraindicated.

* Subdural hematoma: A brain disorder involving a collection of blood in the space between the inner and outer membranes covering the brain. Symptoms usually develop within a short period of time after a head injury. Manual therapy is very intense for such a condition.

* Anticoagulant therapy: Patients who are taking Coumadin (DuPont Pharmaceuticals, Wilmington, Del) or heparin may develop bruises with the application of trigger point therapy. Clearance from the treating physician and consent from the patient should be obtained before application of this technique.

* Advanced osteoporosis: Bone loses calcium and phosphorus, the minerals that make it strong. The tissue becomes less dense and bones become thinner. With sparse tissue or fewer supporting I beams, bones are fragile and fracture easily. It is often called the silent disease because fractures can occur without warning and when they are least expected. If trigger point therapy and stretching exercises are too forceful, fractures may occur.

Communication with the patient's primary care physician, other treating physicians, as well as other clinicians involved in the patient's care is strongly suggested before proceeding with treatment.

REVIEW QUESTIONS

1. In what ways may trigger point and myofascial therapy be harmful to patients with severe advanced osteoporosis?
   A. Local hematoma
   B. Ineffective treatment
   C. Danger of fracture
   D. None of the above

2. A 50-year-old male is suffering from low back pain. Myofascial evaluation reveals active myofascial trigger points on the quadratus lumborum. The patient is on Coumadin. What is the proper intervention?
   A. Trigger point therapy will not help and should not be applied in this case.
   B. Obtain clearance from the physician and consent from the patient before proceeding with treatment.
   C. Obtain clearance from the physician, consent from the patient, and proceed with treatment. Adjust pressure to avoid possible fracture.
   D. Obtain clearance from the physician, consent from the patient, and proceed with treatment. Adjust pressure to avoid bruising.

Chapter 14

PART A REVIEW QUESTIONS ANSWER KEY

CHAPTER 1

1. False
2. True
3. Postisometric relaxation

CHAPTER 2

1. False
2. True
3. 71
4. True
5. True
6. True
7. False

CHAPTER 3

1. False
2. False
3. Accessory
4. True
5. True
6. Actin
7. True
8. False
9. Triad
10. False
11. Motor endplate

12. Motor unit
13. True
14. False
15. True

CHAPTER 4

1. False
2. True
3. False
4. Repetitive movements, high-velocity movements, stress positions
5. True
6. B

CHAPTER 5

1. False
2. False
3. True
4. False
5. False
6. True
7. True
8. False
9. Positive stretch sign
10. B
11. C

Chapter 6

1. True
2. False
3. False

Chapter 7

1. True
2. False
3. False
4. True
5. True
6. Central

Chapter 8

1. False
2. True
3. True

Chapter 9

1. Patient pain recognition
2. False
3. False
4. Active, latent
5. False
6. True
7. True

Chapter 10

1. True
2. False
3. False
4. False
5. True
6. False
7. True
8. True
9. A
10. C

Chapter 11

1. True
2. True
3. False
4. B

Chapter 12

1. True
2. False
3. True
4. False
5. True
6. True

Chapter 13

1. C
2. D

Part B

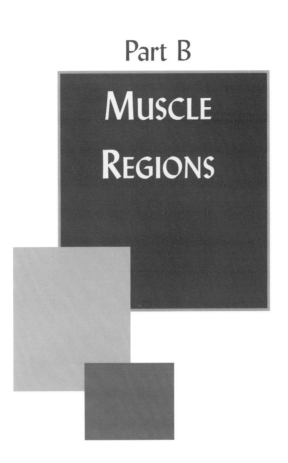

MUSCLE
REGIONS

CERVICAL SPINE REGION

ABBREVIATION LEGEND

RPP	Referred Pain Pattern
TP	Trigger Point
MFS	Myofascial Stretch
PSS	Positive Stretch Sign
HEP	Home Exercise Program
FB	Finger Breadth
HB	Hand Breadth

STERNOCLEIDOMASTOID

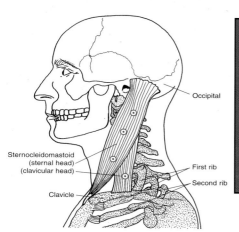

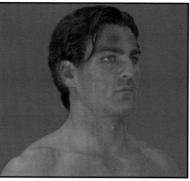

Clavicular

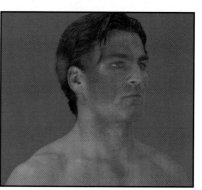

Sternal

ORIGIN

Sternal head—Anterior surface of the manubrium sterni.
Clavicular head—Superior surface of the medial third of the clavicle.

INSERTION

Lateral surface of the mastoid process of the temporal bone and the lateral half of the superior nuchal line of the occiput.

RPP

Occiput (occipital headaches), ear, over the eye and to the cheek, frontal area (frontal headaches), throat, sternum. Occasionally, tinnitus (noise in the ear), blurred vision, and postural dizziness.

TP

Along both divisions of the muscle. Use pincer palpation and avoid contact with the carotid artery and jugular vein.

MFS

Clavicular division: Neck extension, side-bending, and rotation to the opposite side.
Sternal division: Neck extension, side-bending to the opposite side, then rotation to the same side with the muscle stretched.

PSS

Pain at the occipital base and upper cervical spine of the opposite side from the side stretched.

HEP

The patient holds onto a chair or table with the hand to stabilize the shoulder. Follow the MFS above for each of the two SCM divisions.

BIOMECHANICS OF INJURY

Whiplash injury, high-velocity backward neck movement in which the SCM will attempt to control and decelerate movement. Forward neck posture, especially in upper crossed syndrome. Occupations that require constant or repetitive forward neck bending. Improper position of pillow.

CLINICAL NOTES

Usually involved together with scalenii and must be treated together. Correct postural imbalance of the thoracic spine if present.

TRIGGER POINT THERAPY

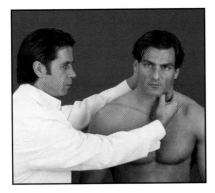 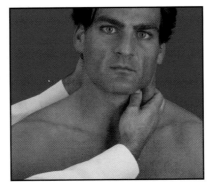 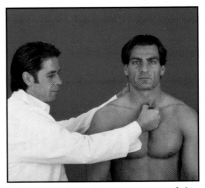

Lower myofascial trigger point of the sternocleidomastoid.

MYOFASCIAL STRETCHES

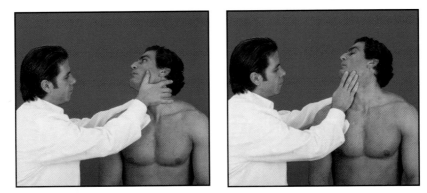

HOME EXERCISE PROGRAM

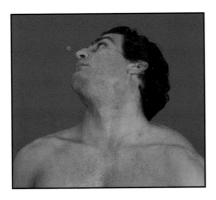 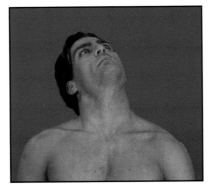 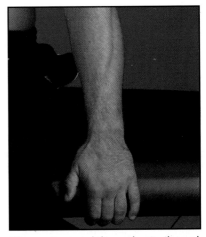

The patient stabilizes the ipsilateral shoulder by holding the table with the hand.

SCALENUS

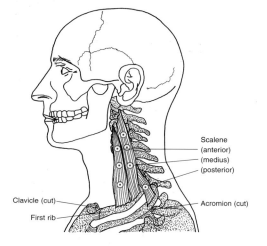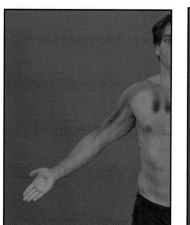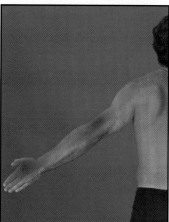

Scalene
(anterior)
(medius)
(posterior)

Clavicle (cut)

First rib

Acromion (cut)

ORIGIN

Medius and anterior—Transverse processes of all cervical vertebrae.
Posterior—Transverse processes of C4, 5, 6.

INSERTION

Medius and anterior—First rib.
Posterior—Second rib.

RPP

Neck, pectoral region, medial border of the scapula, front and back of the arm, radial surface of the forearm, index finger and thumb.

TP

Against transverse processes of cervical vertebrae with flat palpation. Use the thumb or four fingers. Make sure that fingers are behind the SCM muscle. The posterior division may be treated with the thumb.

MFS

Neck side-bending with mild extension. Use the hand to hold onto the chair to stabilize the scapula.

PSS

Pain on the same side of the cervical spine.

HEP

The patient holds onto the chair or table with the hand to stabilize the shoulder. Follow the MFS above.

BIOMECHANICS OF INJURY

Whiplash injury, high-velocity neck movement injuring both the SCM and the SCL. Asthma and other conditions causing difficulty in breathing may cause overshortening of the SCL. Myofascial imbalance will include SCM tightness and SCL laxity resulting in forward neck posture.

CLINICAL NOTES

Usually involved together with SCM and must be treated together. Correct postural imbalance of the thoracic spine if present.

TRIGGER POINT THERAPY

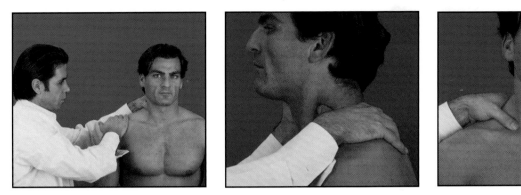

MYOFASCIAL STRETCHES

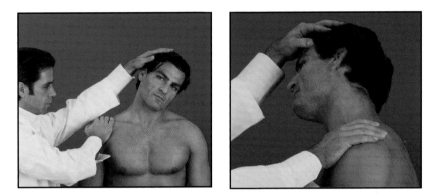

HOME EXERCISE PROGRAM

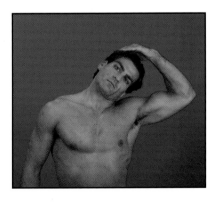

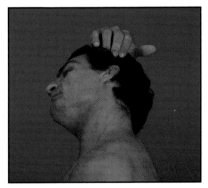

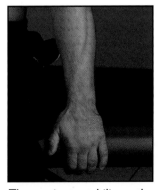

The patient stabilizes the ipsilateral shoulder by holding the table with the hand.

LONGUS COLLI

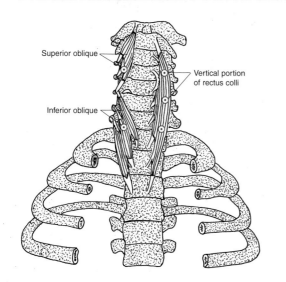

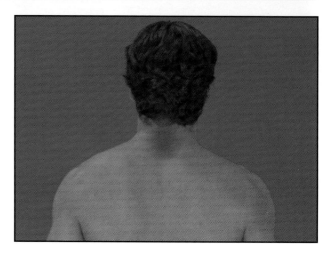

ORIGIN

Third to fifth anterior transverse process of the cervical vertebrae.

INSERTION

Atlas and to the second to fourth anterior vertebral bodies.

RPP

Along the cervical vertebrae and throat.

TP

Along the belly of the muscle with flat, gentle palpation.

MFS

The patient performs a chin tuck while the clinician facilitates midcervical extension.

PSS

Not detected.

HEP

The patient applies the same stretch, bringing the neck to slight extension while maintaining a chin tuck position.

BIOMECHANICS OF INJURY

Overshortening of the SCM and SCL muscles may activate trigger points in the longus colli. Post cervical spine surgery.

CLINICAL NOTES

Extreme caution should be taken when approaching the longus colli muscle from the anterior neck area. Gentle and accurate pressure should be given, avoiding the carotid artery and jugular vein. Have the patient fully relax by breathing out.

TRIGGER POINT THERAPY

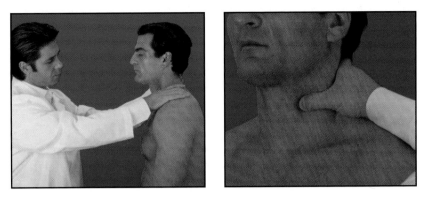

MYOFASCIAL STRETCHES

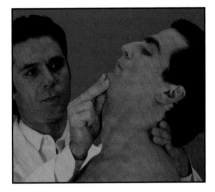

HOME EXERCISE PROGRAM

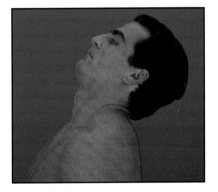

DIGASTRIC

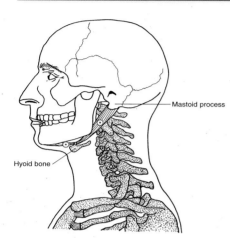

Mastoid process

Hyoid bone

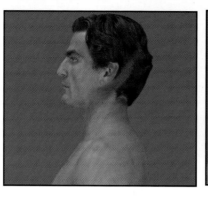 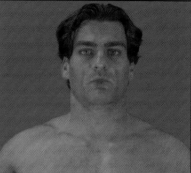

ORIGIN

Anterior—Symphysis of the mandible.
Posterior—Mastoid notch.

INSERTION

Hyoid bone.

RPP

Anterior part refers to the front lower teeth. Posterior part refers to the SCM muscle and its RPP.

TP

Along the belly of the muscle.

MFS

Anterior—Neck extension with the mouth closed.
Posterior—Neck extension and rotation toward the ipsilateral side.

PSS

Pain at the base of the occiput.

HEP

Same as MFS.

BIOMECHANICS OF INJURY

Mandibular movement dysfunction. Sudden movements of the mouth in repetitive sneezing and coughing. Neck hyperextension injuries.

CLINICAL NOTES

Difficulty in swallowing.

TRIGGER POINT THERAPY

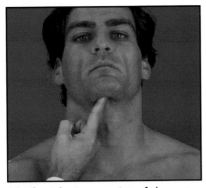

Myofascial trigger point of the anterior division of the digastric muscle.

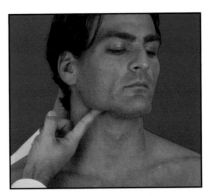

Myofascial trigger point of the posterior division of the digastric muscle.

MYOFASCIAL STRETCHES

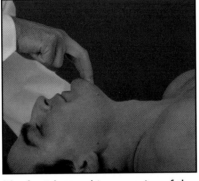

Myofascial stretching exercise of the anterior division of the digastric muscle—neck extension.

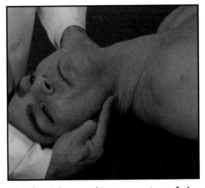

Myofascial stretching exercise of the posterior division of the digastric muscle—neck extension with rotation to the ipsilateral side.

HOME EXERCISE PROGRAM

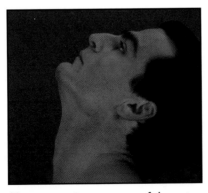

Home exercise program of the anterior division of the digastric muscle—neck extension.

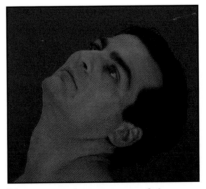

Home exercise program of the posterior division of the digastric muscle—neck extension with rotation to the ipsilateral side.

SUBOCCIPITAL MUSCLES

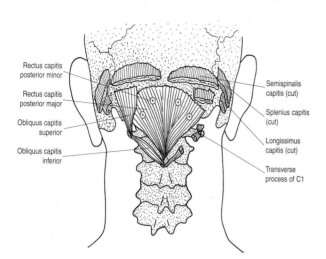

Rectus capitis posterior minor
Rectus capitis posterior major
Obliquus capitis superior
Obliquus capitis inferior
Semispinalis capitis (cut)
Splenius capitis (cut)
Longissimus capitis (cut)
Transverse process of C1

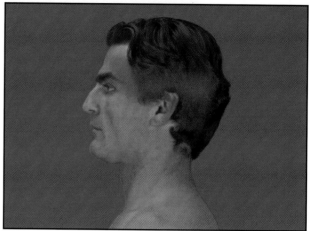

ORIGIN

Occiput, atlas.

INSERTION

Atlas, axis.

RPP

Occipital headaches, deep headaches, pain behind the eye.

TP

Along muscles, suboccipital region.

MFS

Suboccipital decompression technique. Chin tuck followed by upper cervical traction.

PSS

None detected.

HEP

The patient may first perform a chin tuck and then use both hands to provide traction to the upper cervical spine.

BIOMECHANICS OF INJURY

Forward head posture when accommodated by a posterior rotation of the occiput may activate the suboccipital muscles. When the patient is in a prone position for a prolonged time (watching TV or reading a book) and supporting the head with hands under the chin, overshortening of the suboccipital group of muscles may occur. Excessive use of binoculars or eye glasses that need adjustment may cause a compensatory short hyperextension of the neck and further activation of the myofascial trigger points.

CLINICAL NOTES

During the suboccipital decompression technique, the clinician must allow the fingers to relax and apply slow pressure, only as much as allowed by the relaxation of the suboccipital muscles.

TRIGGER POINT THERAPY

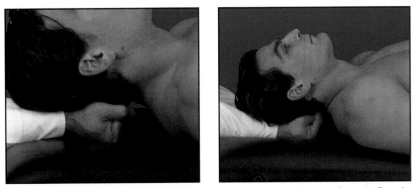

Suboccipital decompression technique is applied in two steps. Step 1: Gentle upward pressure using the fingers into the suboccipital space. Step 2: Gentle traction toward the clinician.

MYOFASCIAL STRETCHES

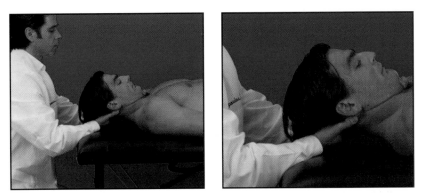

HOME EXERCISE PROGRAM

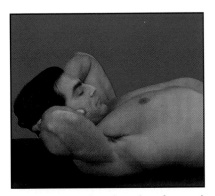 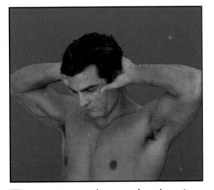 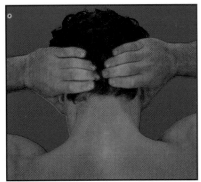

The patient tilts the chin forward (chin tuck) and holds the occiput with the four fingers. The patient then applies forward traction in an anterosuperior direction.

The same stretch can take place in a sitting position.

SPLENIUS CAPITIS AND CERVICIS

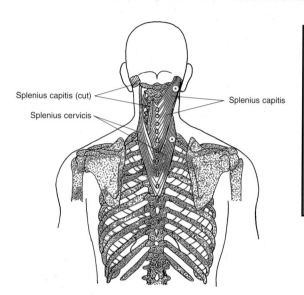

Splenius capitis (cut)
Splenius capitis
Splenius cervicis

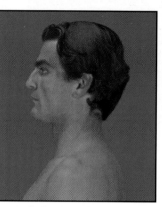

Splenius Capitis

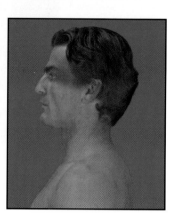

Splenius Cervicis

ORIGIN

Inferior half of the ligamentum nuchae and spinous processes of C7 to T6.

INSERTION

Capitis—Mastoid process and occipital bone.
Cervicis—C3 to C4.

RPP

Top of the head, middle of coronal suture; posterior to the supraorbital margin, neck, and shoulder.

TP

Capitis—Underneath the mastoid process.
Cervicis—Above the angle of the neck lateral to C7.

MFS

Chin tuck with neck flexion and side-bending. The clinician facilitates stretching.

PSS

None detected.

HEP

The patient applies the same stretch using his hand to facilitate movement.

BIOMECHANICS OF INJURY

Postural stress with short repetitive movements of the neck.

TRIGGER POINT THERAPY

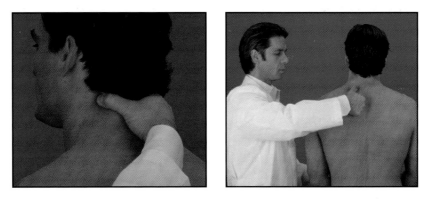

MYOFASCIAL STRETCHES

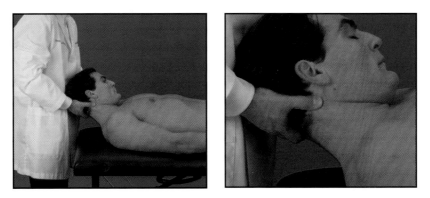

HOME EXERCISE PROGRAM

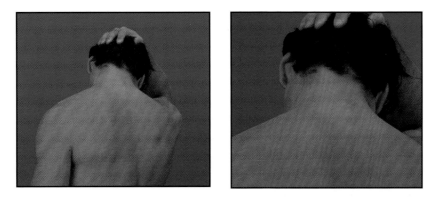

UPPER TRAPEZIUS

ORIGIN

Occipital bone of the ligamentum nuchae.

INSERTION

Outer one-third of the clavicle.

RPP

Posterolateral aspect of the neck, behind the ear, temporal area (temporal headaches) up to the zygoma.

TP

At angle of the neck and shoulder using pincer palpation.

MFS

Neck flexion, side-bending toward the opposite side, and slight rotation toward the ipsilateral side. Give emphasis on side-bending.

PSS

Pain at the opposite side of the neck during stretch.

HEP

The patient is in a sitting position stabilizing the ipsilateral shoulder by holding the underside of the table with the hand. The patient uses the other hand to facilitate neck flexion, side-bending to the opposite side, and rotation to the ipsilateral side. emphasis is placed on side-bending.

BIOMECHANICS OF INJURY

Active overshortening of the muscle when stabilizing a phone handset between the neck and shoulder or carrying heavy bags supported with a belt over the shoulder. Armchairs or wheelchairs with too high arm supports or no supports at all may cause prolonged overstretching or overshortening of the muscle and will activate trigger points.

CLINICAL NOTES

Assess posture of the cervical, thoracolumbar spine, and shoulder. Abnormal posture may cause compensatory tightness of the muscle. Upper crossed syndrome with tight pectoralis muscles may cause activation through overshortening. Stress and anxiety may cause repetitive muscle firing.

TRIGGER POINT THERAPY

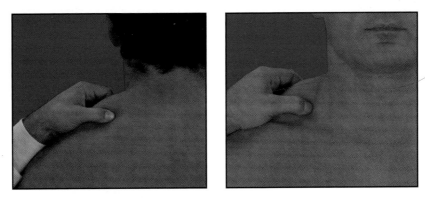

MYOFASCIAL STRETCHES

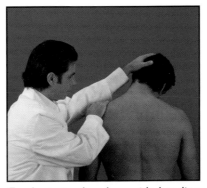

Emphasis is placed on side-bending and rotation to the ipsilateral side.

HOME EXERCISE PROGRAM

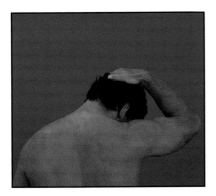
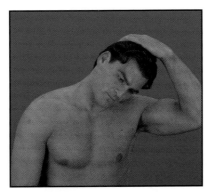
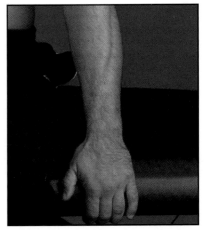

The patient stabilizes the shoulder holding the table with the hand.

LEVATOR SCAPULAE

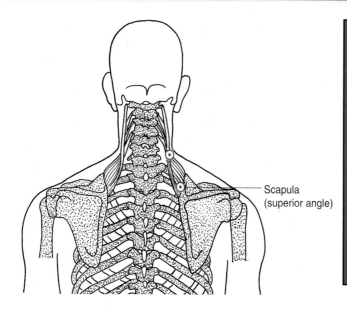

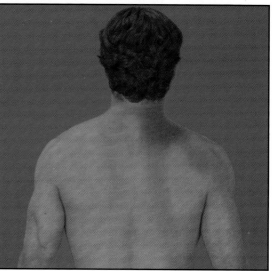

Scapula
(superior angle)

ORIGIN

Transverse processes of C1 to C4.

INSERTION

Vertebral border of scapula above the root of the spine.

RPP

Angle of the neck, along the vertebral border of scapula, posterior shoulder.

TP

Two FB below the angle of the neck and one FB medial.
On the attachments of the muscle to the superior angle of the scapula. Use flat palpation for both points.

MFS

Neck flexion, rotation to the contralateral side, and side-bending to the opposite side with emphasis on flexion.

PSS

Pain in the neck at the opposite side.

HEP

The patient is seated stabilizing the ipsilateral shoulder using the hand under the table. The other hand facilitates neck flexion, rotation, and side-bending to the opposite side. Emphasis is placed on neck flexion.

BIOMECHANICS OF INJURY

Similar activities as in the upper trapezius will activate trigger points of the levator scapulae muscle. Ambulating with canes or crutches that are too long may cause overshortening of the levator scapulae.

CLINICAL NOTES

The clinician must stabilize or even slightly depress the scapula during MFS.

TRIGGER POINT THERAPY

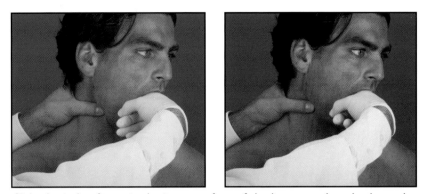

Slide the index finger in the inner surface of the lower teeth and palpate the medial pterygoid behind the last lower molar area.

MYOFASCIAL STRETCHES

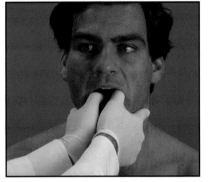

Bilateral stretching of the medial pterygoid muscles.

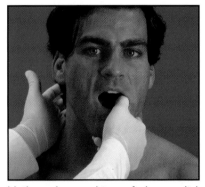

Unilateral stretching of the medial pterygoids. The clinician places the thumb on the lower teeth and the index finger supports the mandible. The clinician performs distraction and anterior glide of the lower jaw.

HOME EXERCISE PROGRAM

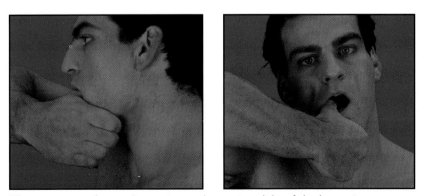

The patient performs distraction and anterior glide of the lower jaw.

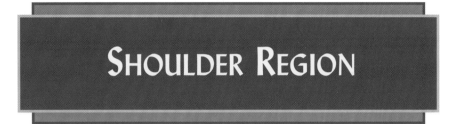

SHOULDER REGION

LATISSIMUS DORSI

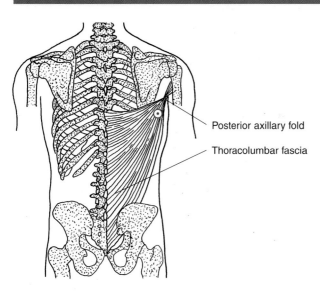

Posterior axillary fold

Thoracolumbar fascia

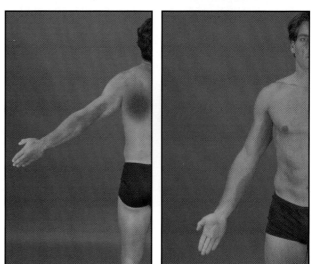

ORIGIN

Spinous process of lower thoracic vertebrae and posterior iliac crest.

INSERTION

Intertubercular groove of the humerus.

RPP

Inferior angle of the scapula; posterior shoulder, arm, forearm, and ulnar aspect of the hand.

TP

Three FB distal to the posterior axillary fold. Use pincer palpation.

MFS

Shoulder abduction to 180 degrees and external rotation.

PSS

Pain at the superior acromion area.

HEP

Stretching the arm in abduction and external rotation against the wall. If a PSS is present during stretch, decrease the degree of abduction.

BIOMECHANICS OF INJURY

Activities that require repetitive extension, adduction, and internal rotation of the shoulder, such as certain types of swimming, may cause activation of trigger points; reaching overhead for objects.

CLINICAL NOTES

During pincer palpation, the clinician must differentiate between the trigger point of the latissimus dorsi and that of the teres major since both are located in approximately the same area. The latissimus dorsi is more lateral and superficial to the teres major.

TRIGGER POINT THERAPY

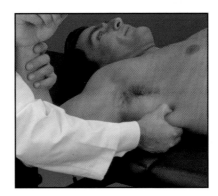

MYOFASCIAL STRETCHES

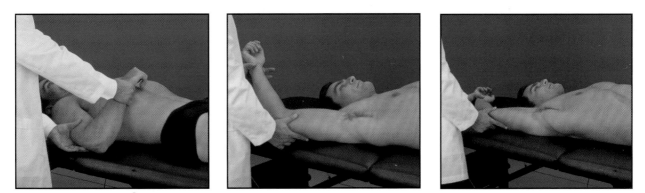

HOME EXERCISE PROGRAM

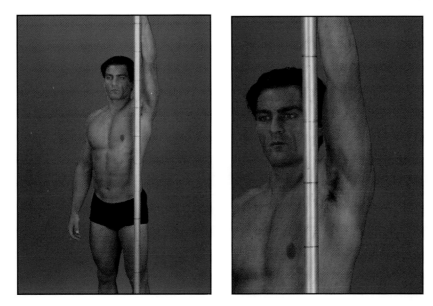

TERES MAJOR

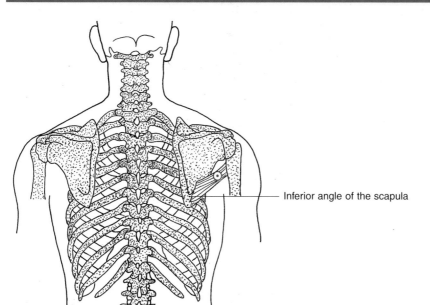

Inferior angle of the scapula

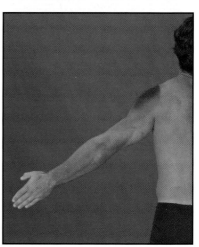

ORIGIN

Inferior angle of the scapula.

INSERTION

Posterior bicipital ridge.

RPP

Posterior deltoid region and forearm.

TP

Three FB above the inferior angle of the scapula along the lateral border. Use pincer palpation.

MFS

Hyperabduction of the shoulder and external rotation.

PSS

Pain at the superior acromion area.

HEP

Stretching the arm in hyperabduction, external rotation against the wall. If a PSS is present during stretch, decrease the degree of abduction.

BIOMECHANICS OF INJURY

Similar to the latissimus dorsi.

CLINICAL NOTES

During pincer palpation, the clinician must differentiate between the trigger point of the teres major and that of the latissimus dorsi since both are located in approximately the same area.

TRIGGER POINT THERAPY

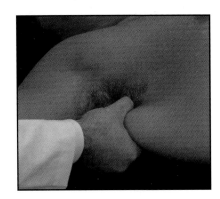

MYOFASCIAL STRETCHES

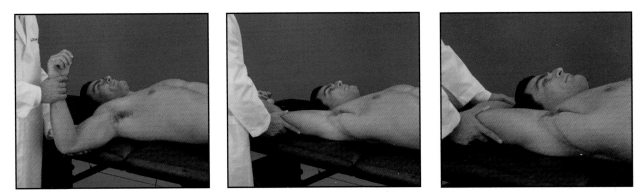

HOME EXERCISE PROGRAM

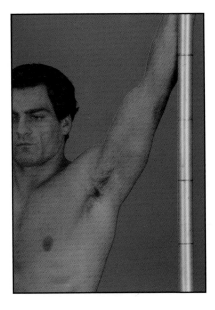

SUBSCAPULARIS

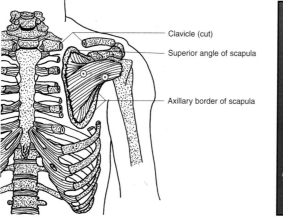

Clavicle (cut)

Superior angle of scapula

Axillary border of scapula

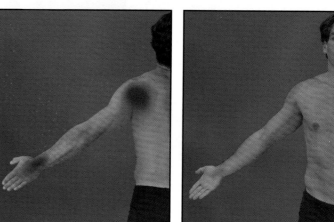

ORIGIN

Subscapular fossa on the costal surface of the scapula.

INSERTION

Lesser tubercle of the humerus. Its tendon is attached to the fibrous capsule of the shoulder joint.

RPP

Posterior deltoid area, scapula, posterior arm, wrist; occasionally on the anterior shoulder and palmar surface of the wrist.

TP

Subscapular fossa along the axillary border and toward the superior angle of the scapula. Use flat palpation with four fingers in medial-superior and posterior directions. Scapular depression or traction of the arm may facilitate reaching for the trigger points.

MFS

Arm external rotation and abduction to 180 degrees. If a PSS is present, adjust shoulder abduction with shoulder flexion and progressively move to abduction.

PSS

Pain at the superior acromion area.

HEP

Stretching the arm in abduction and external rotation against the wall. Progress the patient to various degrees of shoulder flexion starting from 140 to 180 degrees of flexion-abduction, external rotation. If a PSS is present during stretch, decrease degrees of flexion.

BIOMECHANICS OF INJURY

Most shoulder injuries will involve the subscapularis muscle, as it is a main stabilizer of the scapula. Frozen shoulder, as well as other shoulder pathologies with limitation of shoulder abduction, may involve the subscapularis muscle. Throwing activities may result in high-velocity injury to the muscle. Dislocation of the shoulder and prolonged immobilization may cause microtrauma of the subscapularis.

CLINICAL NOTES

Subscapularis myofascial involvement will affect the scapulohumeral rhythm and will cause abnormal shoulder mechanics during movement. The infraspinatus muscle may also be myofascially involved.

TRIGGER POINT THERAPY

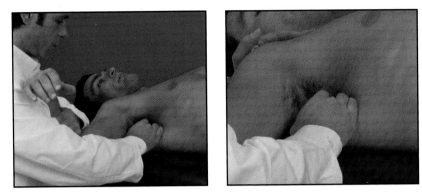

MYOFASCIAL STRETCHES

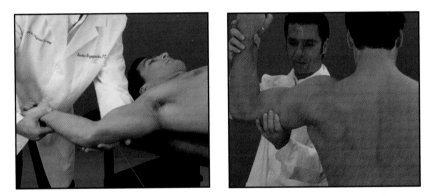

HOME EXERCISE PROGRAM

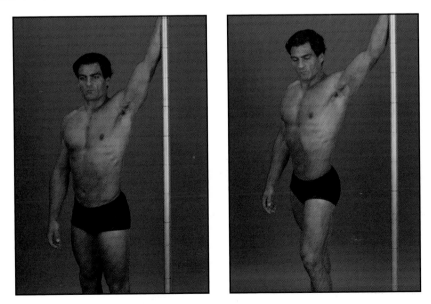

SUPRASPINATUS

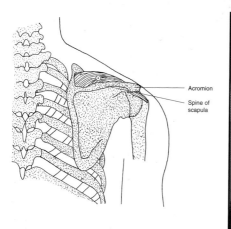

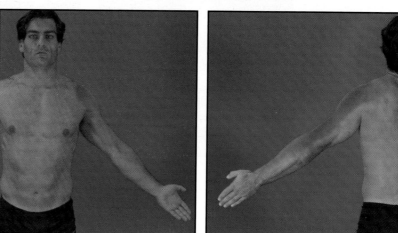

ORIGIN

Supraspinous fossa of the scapula.

INSERTION

The greater tuberosity of the humerus.

RPP

Mid-deltoid region of the humerus, arm, lateral epicondyle.

TP

One FB above the middle of the spine of the scapula and in the space between the scapula and the clavicle, medial to the acromion.

MFS

Internal rotation of the shoulder. Internal rotation and horizontal adduction from a lower position.

PSS

Pain at the anterior acromion area.

HEP

Stretching the arm in internal rotation and horizontal adduction, facilitating stretch with the other hand.

BIOMECHANICS OF INJURY

Lifting and carrying heavy objects and prolonged overhead activities.

TRIGGER POINT THERAPY

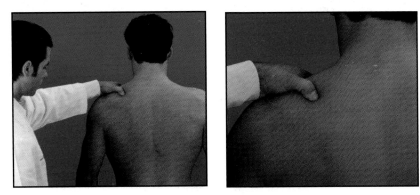

MYOFASCIAL STRETCHES

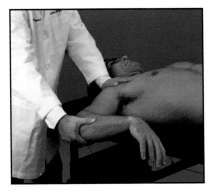

HOME EXERCISE PROGRAM

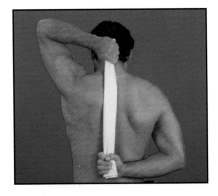 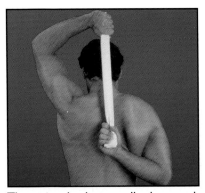

The uninvolved arm pulls the towel cephalad and facilitates stretching of the involved muscle.

INFRASPINATUS

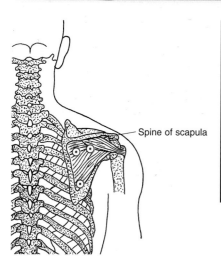

Spine of scapula

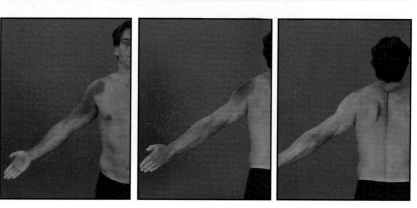

ORIGIN

Infraspinous fossa of the scapula.

INSERTION

Greater tuberosity of the humerus.

RPP

Anterior deltoid region, shoulder joint, medial border of the scapula, front and lateral aspects of the arm and forearm.

TP

Two FB below the medial portion of the spine of the scapula. Three FB above the inferior angle of the scapula. Use flat palpation.

MFS

Internal rotation of the shoulder. Internal rotation and horizontal adduction from a higher position.

PSS

Pain at the anterior acromion area.

HEP

Stretch the arm in internal rotation and horizontal adduction from a higher position.

BIOMECHANICS OF INJURY

Activities that involve repetitive or high-velocity internal rotation movements.

CLINICAL NOTES

Female patients may complain of pain when trying to button a skirt or bra. Use the hand to shoulder blade test to assess. Internal rotation of the shoulder when reaching toward the contralateral scapula.

TRIGGER POINT THERAPY

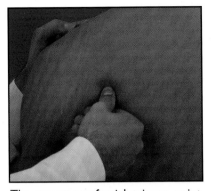

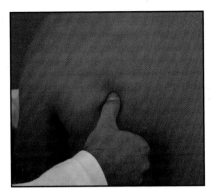

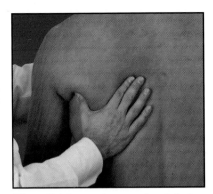

The upper myofascial trigger point of the infraspinatus muscle.

The lower myofascial trigger point of the infraspinatus muscle.

The clinician palpates the inferior angle of the scapula.

MYOFASCIAL STRETCHES

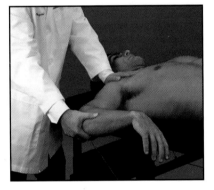

HOME EXERCISE PROGRAM

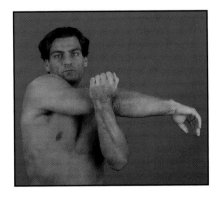

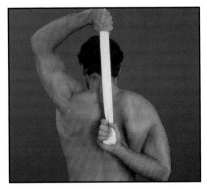

The uninvolved arm pulls the towel cephalad and facilitates stretching of the involved muscle.

PECTORALIS MAJOR

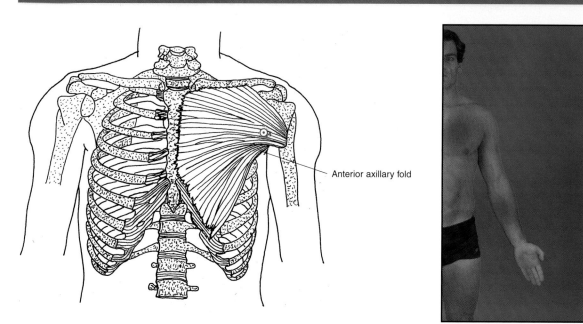

Anterior axillary fold

ORIGIN

Clavicle, sternum, and cartilages of the first six ribs.

INSERTION

Greater tubercle of the humerus.

RPP

Chest, breast, shoulder, and medial arm and forearm.

TP

Anterior axillary fold. Use pincer palpation.

MFS

The patient abducts the shoulder to 90 degrees and flexes the elbow to 90 degrees. The clinician facilitates horizontal abduction from this position.

PSS

Pain at the posterior acromion area.

HEP

The patient stands by a door and positions the shoulder to 90 degrees abduction and 90 degrees elbow flexion. He then leans anteriorly (horizontal abduction) while supporting the forearm and hand at the open doorway.

BIOMECHANICS OF INJURY

Upper crossed syndrome with rounded shoulders and tightness of the pectoralis muscle. Prolonged sitting and heavy lifting of weights. Asthma and other respiratory conditions when shallow breathing is present.

CLINICAL NOTES

Pectoralis major involvement may activate myofascial trigger points on the pectoralis minor.

TRIGGER POINT THERAPY

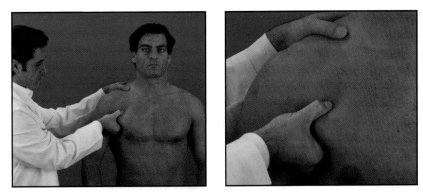

MYOFASCIAL STRETCHES

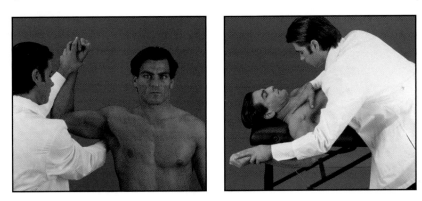

HOME EXERCISE PROGRAM

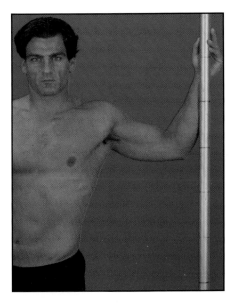

PECTORALIS MINOR

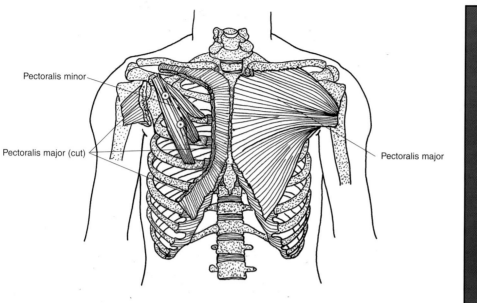

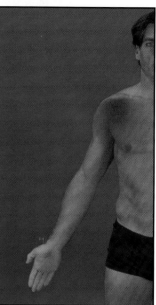

ORIGIN

Anterior surface of the third to fifth ribs.

INSERTION

Coracoid process of the scapula.

RPP

Upper chest area, anterior shoulder, medial aspect of the arm.

TP

In the midclavicular line down to the third rib. Two to three FB below the lateral third of the clavicle.

MFS

Abduction of the shoulder to 120 degrees and then horizontal abduction. The clinician facilitates shoulder movement.

PSS

Pain in the posterior acromion area.

HEP

The patient stands by a door and positions the shoulder to 120 degrees of abduction. He then leans anteriorly (horizontal abduction) while supporting the forearm and hand at the open doorway.

BIOMECHANICS OF INJURY

Same as the pectoralis major.

TRIGGER POINT THERAPY

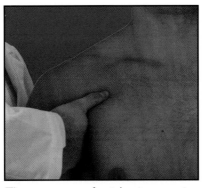
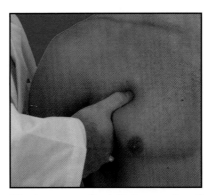

The upper myofascial trigger point of the pectoralis minor muscle.

The lower myofascial trigger point of the pectoralis minor muscle.

MYOFASCIAL STRETCHES

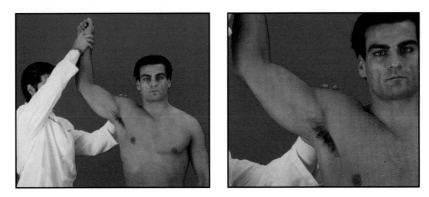

HOME EXERCISE PROGRAM

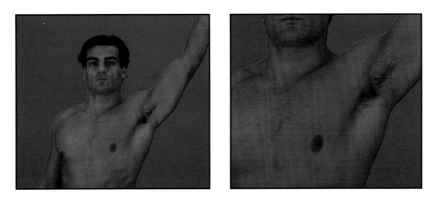

DELTOID

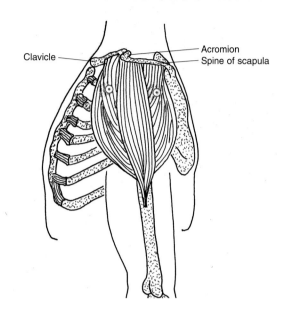

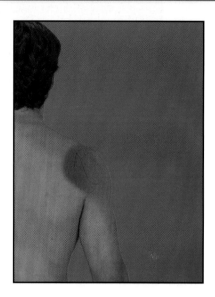

ORIGIN

Anterior—Lateral third of the anterior and superior surfaces of the clavicle.
Posterior—The spine of the scapula.

INSERTION

Deltoid tubercle of the humerus.

RPP

Locally on the muscle; shoulder.

TP

Anterior—Three FB below the anterior margin of the acromion.
Posterior—Two FB caudal to the posterior margin of the acromion.
Use flat palpation.

MFS

Anterior—Shoulder extension with elbow extension and neutral position of the forearm.
Posterior—Shoulder horizontal adduction from a higher position and elbow flexed.
The clinician facilitates stretch.

PSS

Pain at the superior acromion area.

HEP

Same as MFS.

BIOMECHANICS OF INJURY

High-velocity injuries in sports activities. Direct trauma.

TRIGGER POINT THERAPY

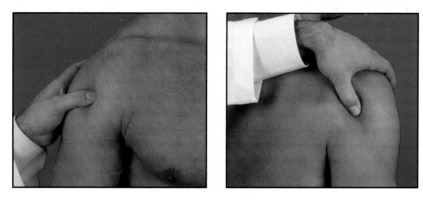

MYOFASCIAL STRETCHES

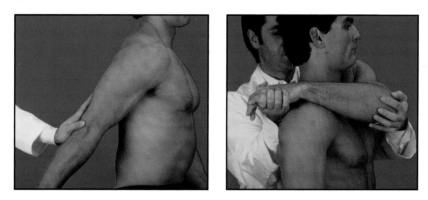

HOME EXERCISE PROGRAM

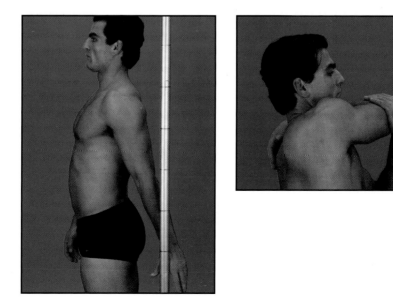

SUBCLAVIUS

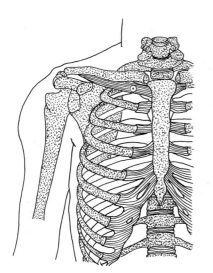
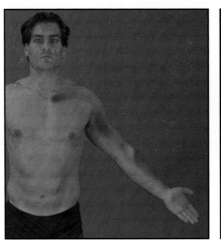
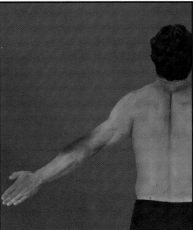

ORIGIN

First rib.

INSERTION

Middle third of the clavicle.

RPP

Clavicular area; biceps and forearm area.

TP

Two FB lateral to the sternum at the sternoclavicular junction.

MFS

Shoulder moves to 180 degrees of flexion as the clinician facilitates upward rotation of the clavicle.

PSS

None detected.

HEP

None.

BIOMECHANICS OF INJURY

Direct trauma, clavicular fracture.

CLINICAL NOTES

The clinician should be very gentle when facilitating the upward rotation of the clavicle.

TRIGGER POINT THERAPY

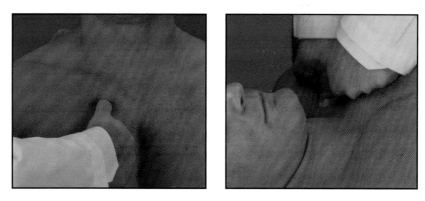

MYOFASCIAL STRETCHES

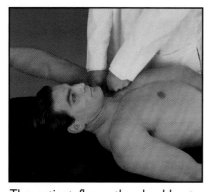

The patient flexes the shoulder to 180 degrees and the clavicle rotates upward.

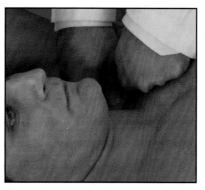

The clinician facilitates clavicular rotation.

STERNALIS

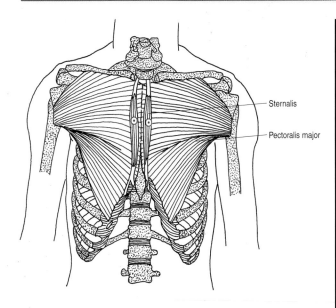

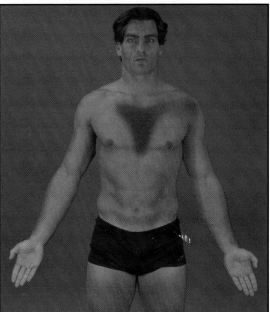

Sternalis

Pectoralis major

ORIGIN

Parallel to the sternum in one or both sides in only 5% of the population.

INSERTION

Sternum.

RPP

Sternum, superior chest area, and medial arm.

TP

Several possible points, one FB lateral to the body of the sternum.

MFS

None.

PSS

None detected.

HEP

None.

BIOMECHANICS OF INJURY

None.

TRIGGER POINT THERAPY

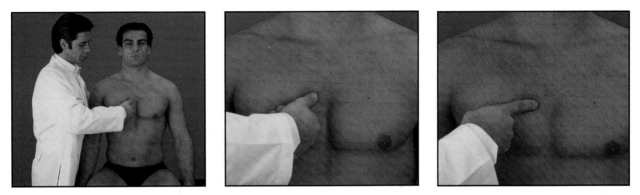

MYOFASCIAL STRETCHES

You may perform only trigger point palpation. No myofascial stretching exercises are applicable.

UPPER EXTREMITY REGION

Biceps Brachii

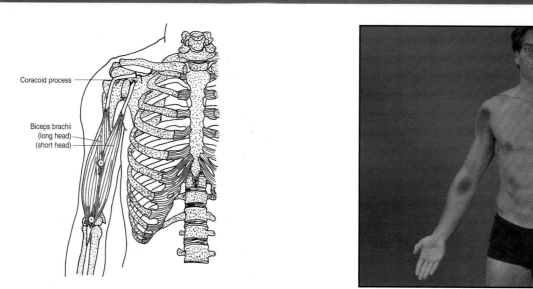

Coracoid process

Biceps brachii
(long head)
(short head)

ORIGIN

Long head—Supraglenoid tuberosity of the scapula.
Short head—Coracoid process of the scapula.

INSERTION

Tuberosity of the radius.

RPP

Along the muscle toward the suprascapular region; near the insertion of the muscle.

TP

Belly of the muscle in the midarm, and three FB above the insertion of the muscle.

MFS

Extension of the elbow with the shoulder extended. The clinician facilitates the stretch.

PSS

Pain at the elbow area.

HEP

Same as MFS. The patient may use the doorknob to facilitate stretch.

BIOMECHANICS OF INJURY

Sudden overstretching of the muscle, sports activities, lifting heavy objects. In cases of elbow fractures when prolonged immobilization is required, trigger points may be activated through prolonged overshortening.

CLINICAL NOTES

Pincer palpation is recommended for the middle trigger point and flat palpation for the lower one.
Use the lower trigger point combined with a postisometric relaxation technique for limitations of elbow extension after prolonged immobilization and post fractures. The clinician may take advantage of the fact that the long head of the biceps crosses the shoulder, and shoulder extension will stretch the proximal biceps muscle.

TRIGGER POINT THERAPY

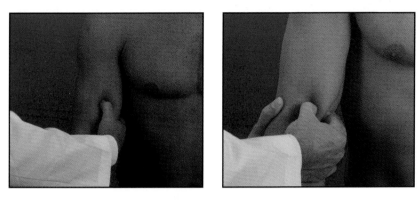

MYOFASCIAL STRETCHES

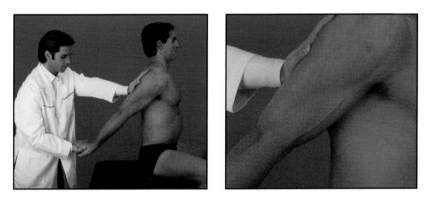

HOME EXERCISE PROGRAM

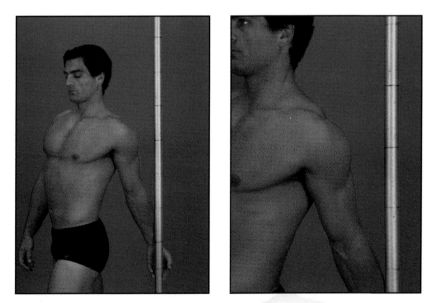

TRICEPS

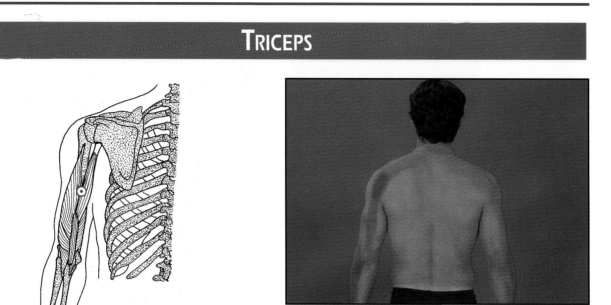

ORIGIN

Lateral head—Humeral groove.
Long head—Infraglenoid tuberosity of the scapula.
Medial head—Shaft of the humerus.

INSERTION

Olecranon process.

RPP

Posterior aspect of the arm, medial and lateral epicondyle, fingers.

TP

Belly of the muscle in midarm. Use pincer palpation.

MFS

Shoulder flexion and complete elbow flexion. The clinician facilitates elbow flexion.

PSS

Pain in the elbow joint.

HEP

Same as MFS. The patient may use the other hand to facilitate stretch.

BIOMECHANICS OF INJURY

Sudden overstretching of the muscle, sports activities, lifting heavy objects.

CLINICAL NOTES

Entrapment of the radial nerve may occur from tightness in the lateral head.

TRIGGER POINT THERAPY

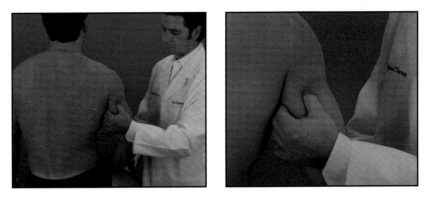

MYOFASCIAL STRETCHES

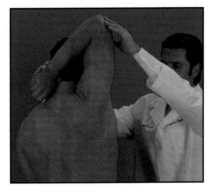

HOME EXERCISE PROGRAM

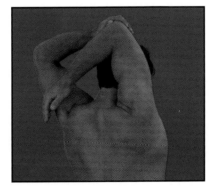

BRACHIORADIALIS

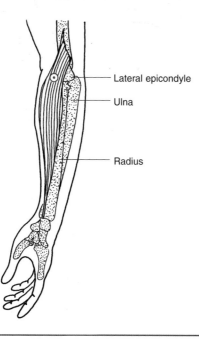

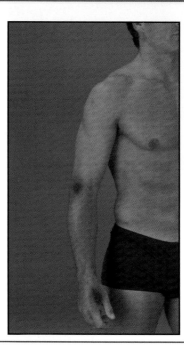

Lateral epicondyle

Ulna

Radius

ORIGIN

Supracondylar area of the lateral aspect of the humerus.

INSERTION

Above the styloid process.

RPP

Lateral epicondyle, along the muscle, and web space.

TP

One FB below the flexor crease and midway between the biceps tendon and lateral epicondyle. Use pincer or flat palpation.

MFS

Elbow extension and pronation. Palmar flexion, ulnar deviation with emphasis on palmar flexion. The clinician facilitates the wrist movement. If a PSS is present, decrease the degree of ulnar deviation.

PSS

Pain at the ulnar wrist area.

HEP

As MFS above with the patient using the other hand to facilitate stretch.

BIOMECHANICS OF INJURY

Sports activities, especially when wrist extension is required from a pronated position.

CLINICAL NOTES

The muscle can be involved in cases of "tennis elbow."

TRIGGER POINT THERAPY

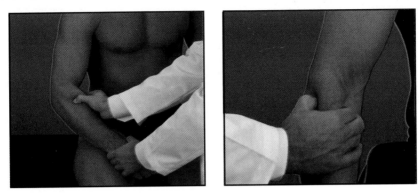

MYOFASCIAL STRETCHES

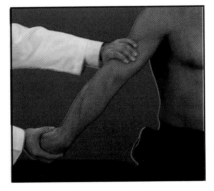

HOME EXERCISE PROGRAM

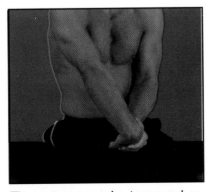
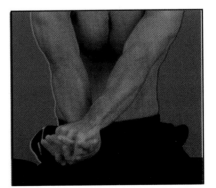

The patient must be instructed to maintain full elbow extension.

SUPINATOR

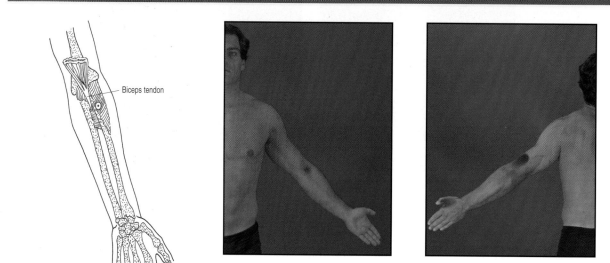

Biceps tendon

ORIGIN

Lateral epicondyle of the humerus.

INSERTION

Upper third of the radial shaft.

RPP

Lateral epicondyle, forearm, and web space.

TP

Radial to the most distal part of the insertion of the biceps tendon. Use flat palpation aiming toward the head of the radius.

MFS

Elbow extension and pronation. Palmar flexion of the wrist and ulnar deviation with emphasis on ulnar deviation and pronation. If the PSS is present, decrease the degree of ulnar deviation.

PSS

Pain at the ulnar wrist area.

HEP

As above with the patient using the other hand to facilitate stretch.

BIOMECHANICS OF INJURY

Sports activities, especially when supination is required. Repetitive supination when the elbow is extended may activate trigger points.

CLINICAL NOTES

The muscle can be involved in cases of "tennis elbow." Entrapment of the deep branch of the radial nerve at the arcade of Frohse may occur. Check for weakness of the extensors. The supinator will be spared.

TRIGGER POINT THERAPY

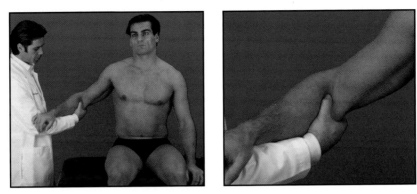

MYOFASCIAL STRETCHES

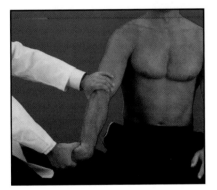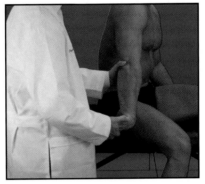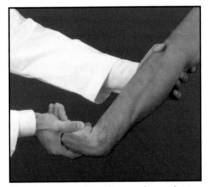

Emphasis is placed on ulnar deviation and pronation.

HOME EXERCISE PROGRAM

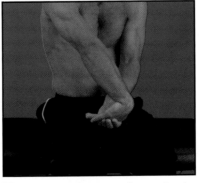

The patient is instructed to maintain the elbow in full extension.

PRONATOR TERES

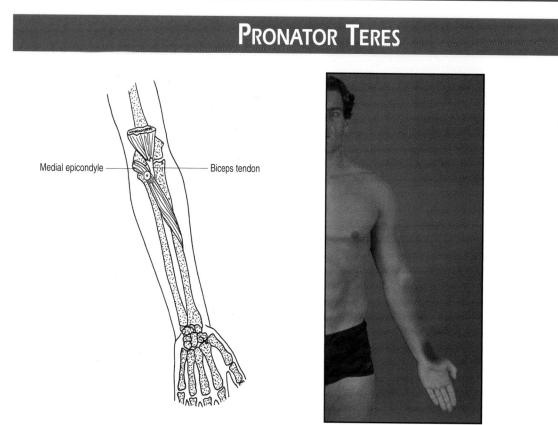

Medial epicondyle ——   —— Biceps tendon

ORIGIN

Medial epicondyle of the humerus and coronoid process of the ulna.

INSERTION

Lateral surface of the radius at the midshaft.

RPP

Radial side of the wrist and anterior surface of the forearm.

TP

Two FB distal to the midpoint of a line connecting the medial epicondyle and biceps tendon. Use flat palpation.

MFS

Elbow extension and complete supination; wrist extension will facilitate further supination. The clinician handles the wrist. The elbow must be extended.

PSS

Not detected.

HEP

As MFS above with the patient using the other hand to facilitate wrist extension and supination.

BIOMECHANICS OF INJURY

Sports activities; wrist and elbow fractures may activate myofascial trigger points.

TRIGGER POINT THERAPY

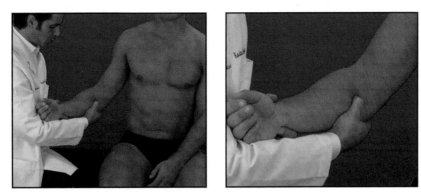

MYOFASCIAL STRETCHES

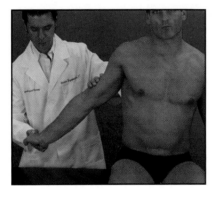
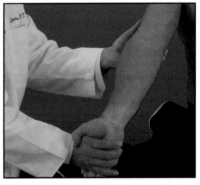

During the myofascial stretch, the elbow must be in full extension.

HOME EXERCISE PROGRAM

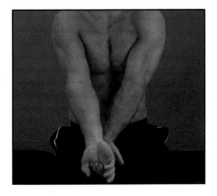

FLEXOR CARPI ULNARIS

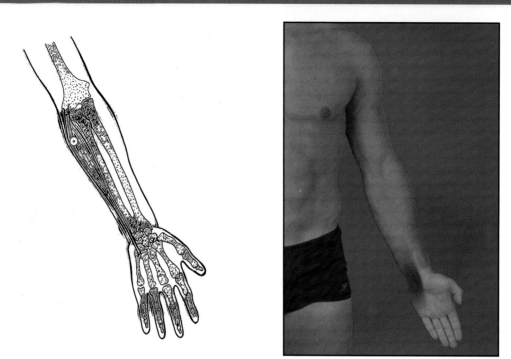

ORIGIN

Medial epicondyle of the humerus; medial margin of the olecranon.

INSERTION

Pisiform, hamate, and fifth metacarpal.

RPP

Ulnar side of the wrist.

TP

Two to three FB below the flexor crease of the elbow, medial to the ulnar side. Flat palpation.

MFS

Elbow extension, supination, wrist extension, and radial deviation, with emphasis on radial deviation.

PSS

Pain at the radial wrist area.

HEP

As MFS above with the patient using the other hand to facilitate stretch.

BIOMECHANICS OF INJURY

Tight grip of larger objects may activate trigger points in the muscle.

CLINICAL NOTES

All wrist and finger flexor muscles may participate in the "trigger finger" mechanism either directly or indirectly.

TRIGGER POINT THERAPY

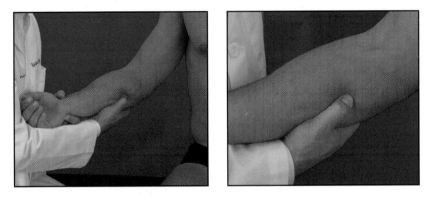

MYOFASCIAL STRETCHES

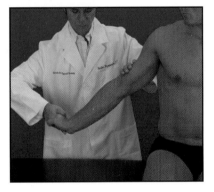

HOME EXERCISE PROGRAM

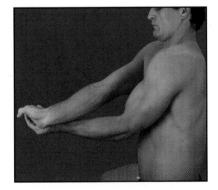

FLEXOR CARPI RADIALIS

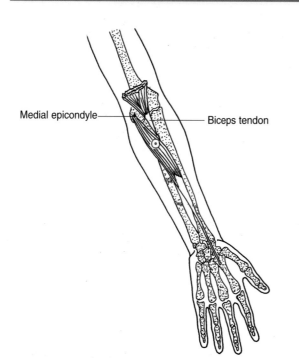

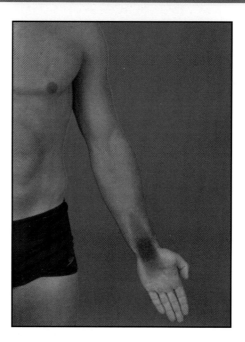

Medial epicondyle ———   ——— Biceps tendon

ORIGIN

Medial epicondyle of the humerus.

INSERTION

Base of the second metacarpal.

RPP

Radial and anterior sides of the wrist.

TP

Three to four FB below the midline connecting the medial epicondyle and biceps tendon. Use flat palpation.

MFS

Elbow extension, supination, wrist extension, and radial deviation, with emphasis on wrist extension and supination.

PSS

Pain at the posterior carpal area.

HEP

As above with the patient using the other hand to facilitate extension of the wrist and supination.

BIOMECHANICS OF INJURY

Repetitive finger and wrist motion, such as with assembly line workers, cashiers, etc.

TRIGGER POINT THERAPY

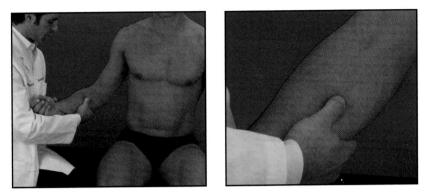

MYOFASCIAL STRETCHES

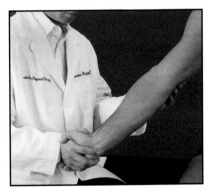

HOME EXERCISE PROGRAM

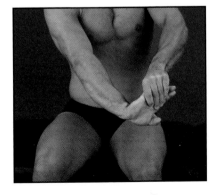

EXTENSOR CARPI RADIALIS (LONGUS AND BREVIS)

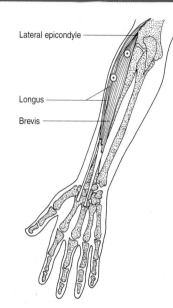

Lateral epicondyle

Longus

Brevis

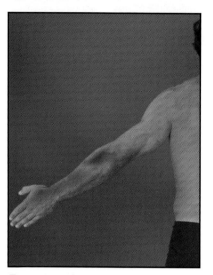

Extensor Carpi Radialis Longus

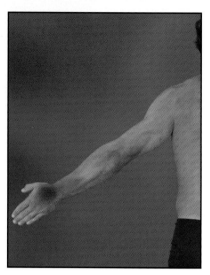

Extensor Carpi Radialis Brevis

ORIGIN

Longus—Lower one-third of the supracondylar ridge of the humerus.
Brevis—Lateral epicondyle of the humerus.

INSERTION

Longus—Dorsal surface of the base of the second metacarpal.
Brevis—Dorsal surface of the base of the third metacarpal.

RPP

Wrist, web space, lateral epicondyle, forearm.

TP

Two FB distal to the lateral epicondyle with flat palpation.

MFS

Elbow extension, pronation, and palmar flexion of the wrist. The clinician facilitates the wrist movement.

PSS

Pain in the palmar aspect of the wrist.

HEP

The patient applies the same stretch using the other hand to facilitate wrist movement.

BIOMECHANICS OF INJURY

Activities that require prolonged or repetitive extension of the wrist, as in typing or various sports activities like tennis and golf.

CLINICAL NOTES

Due to the fact that there are several trigger points of other muscles in the same area, the clinician must ask the patient to actively contract the muscle in order to properly identify it.

TRIGGER POINT THERAPY

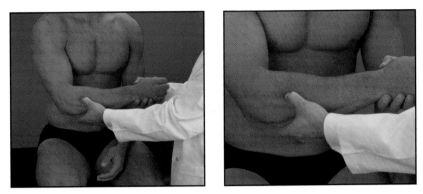

MYOFASCIAL STRETCHES

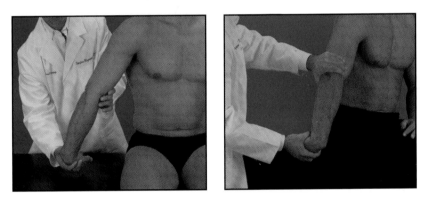

HOME EXERCISE PROGRAM

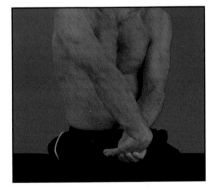

EXTENSOR CARPI ULNARIS

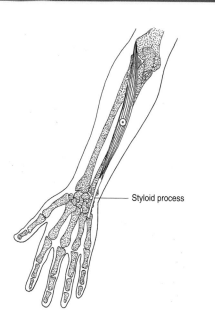

Styloid process

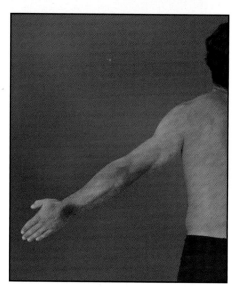

ORIGIN

Lateral epicondyle of the humerus.

INSERTION

Dorsal surface of the base of the fifth metacarpal.

RPP

Ulnar and anterior sides of the wrist.

TP

Midpoint of the ulna, one FB medial from the shaft of the ulna. Flat palpation.

MFS

Elbow extension, pronation, and palmar flexion of the wrist. The clinician facilitates the wrist movement.

PSS

Pain in the palmar aspect of the wrist.

HEP

The patient applies the same stretch using the other hand to facilitate wrist movement.

BIOMECHANICS OF INJURY

Activities that require prolonged or repetitive extension of the wrist, as in typing or various sports activities like tennis and golf.

CLINICAL NOTES

Due to the fact that there are several trigger points of other muscles in the same area, the clinician must ask the patient to actively contract the muscle in order to properly identify it.

TRIGGER POINT THERAPY

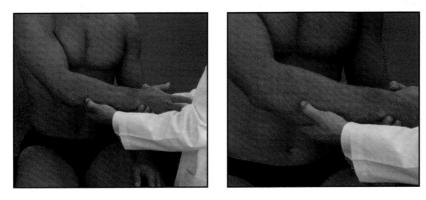

MYOFASCIAL STRETCHES

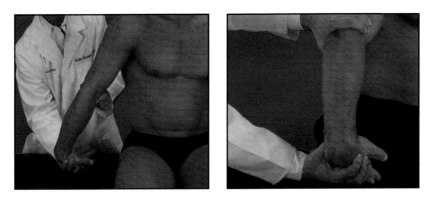

HOME EXERCISE PROGRAM

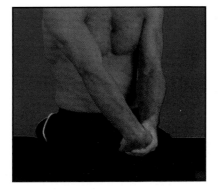

EXTENSOR DIGITORUM

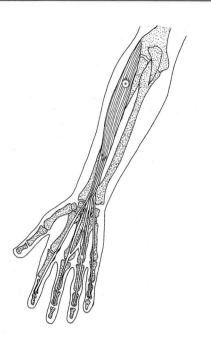

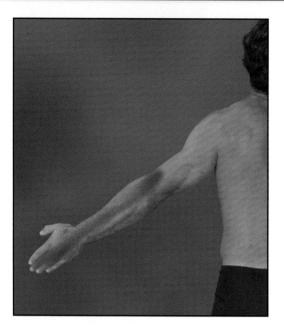

ORIGIN

Lateral epicondyle of the humerus.

INSERTION

Dorsal surface of the base of the second to fifth phalanges.

RPP

Middle finger, forearm, and lateral epicondyle.

TP

Four FB below the lateral epicondyle.

MFS

Elbow extension, pronation, palmar flexion of the wrist, and flexion of the fingers. Emphasis should be given on flexion of the fingers.

PSS

Pain in the palmar aspect of the wrist.

HEP

The patient applies the same stretch using the other hand to facilitate finger flexion movement.

BIOMECHANICS OF INJURY

Activities that require prolonged or repetitive movement of the fingers, such as with musicians and typists.

CLINICAL NOTES

Due to the fact that there are several trigger points of other muscles in the same area, the clinician must ask the patient to actively contract the muscle in order to properly identify it.

TRIGGER POINT THERAPY

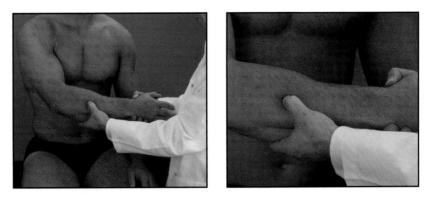

MYOFASCIAL STRETCHES

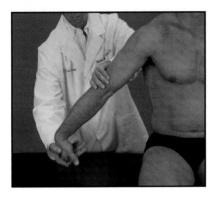
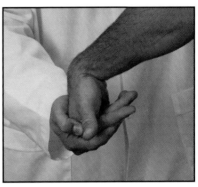

Emphasis is placed on finger flexion.

HOME EXERCISE PROGRAM

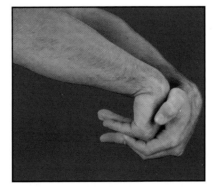

EXTENSOR INDICIS PROPRIUS

ORIGIN

Dorsal surface of the lower half of the ulnar shaft.

INSERTION

Index finger.

RPP

Volar aspect of the wrist and hand.

TP

Two FB proximal to the ulnar styloid in the interspace between the ulna and radius.

MFS

Palmar flexion of the wrist and flexion of the index finger. The clinician facilitates the finger movement.

PSS

Not detected.

HEP

The patient applies the same stretch using the other hand to facilitate finger movement.

BIOMECHANICS OF INJURY

Direct flexor trauma of the index finger may cause overstretching injury. Repetitive motion in daily or work activities may result in trigger point formation.

TRIGGER POINT THERAPY

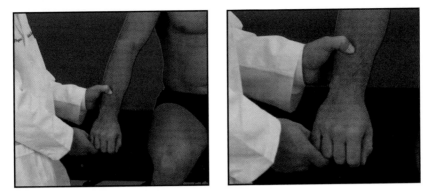

MYOFASCIAL STRETCHES

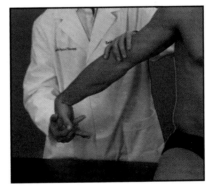

HOME EXERCISE PROGRAM

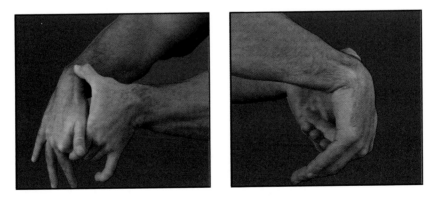

ABDUCTOR POLLICIS BREVIS

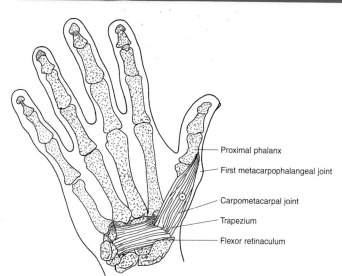

Proximal phalanx
First metacarpophalangeal joint
Carpometacarpal joint
Trapezium
Flexor retinaculum

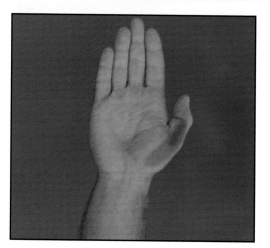

ORIGIN
Scaphoid and trapezium.

INSERTION
Proximal phalanx of the thumb.

RPP
Radial and palmar aspects of the thumb.

TP
Midline of the first metacarpophalangeal joint of the thumb and the carpometacarpal joint. Flat palpation.

MFS
Extension of the thumb followed by adduction.

PSS
Pain at the first metacarpophalangeal joint.

HEP
As MFS above with the patient using the other thumb and fingers to facilitate stretch.

BIOMECHANICS OF INJURY
Handling, holding, and grasping small objects for a prolonged time. Writing and painting activities will affect all thenar muscles.

CLINICAL NOTES
All thenar muscles may participate in a "trigger thumb" condition.

TRIGGER POINT THERAPY

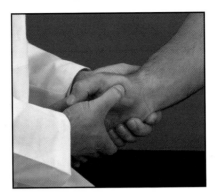

MYOFASCIAL STRETCHES

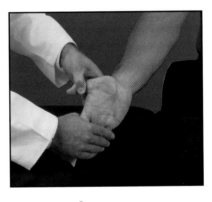

HOME EXERCISE PROGRAM

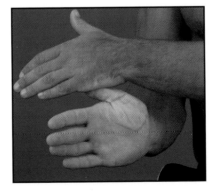

FLEXOR POLLICIS BREVIS

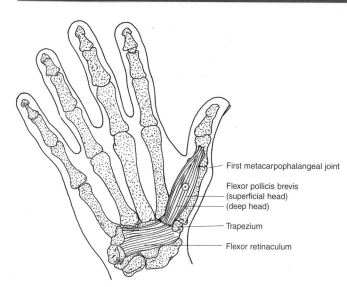

First metacarpophalangeal joint

Flexor pollicis brevis
(superficial head)
(deep head)

Trapezium

Flexor retinaculum

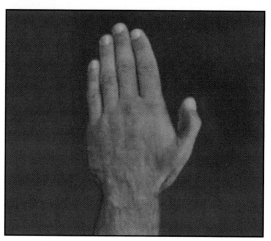

ORIGIN

Superficial head—Trapezium and flexor retinaculum.
Deep head—Ulnar side of first metacarpal.

INSERTION

Superficial head—Radial side of the base of the proximal phalanx of the thumb.

RPP

Palmar aspect of thumb.

TP

Midline between the origin and insertion. Flat palpation.

MFS

Extension of the thumb.

PSS

Pain at the first metacarpophalangeal joint.

HEP

As above with the patient using the other thumb and fingers to facilitate stretch.

BIOMECHANICS OF INJURY

See abductor pollicis brevis.

CLINICAL NOTES

All thenar muscles may participate in a "trigger thumb" condition.

TRIGGER POINT THERAPY

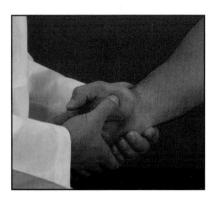

MYOFASCIAL STRETCHES

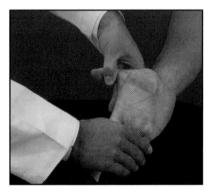

HOME EXERCISE PROGRAM

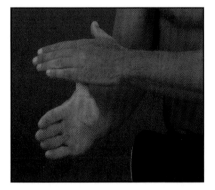

ADDUCTOR POLLICIS

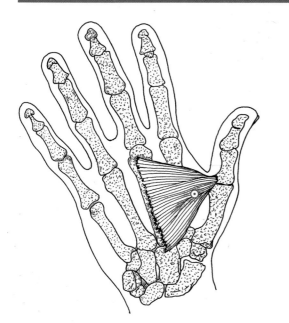
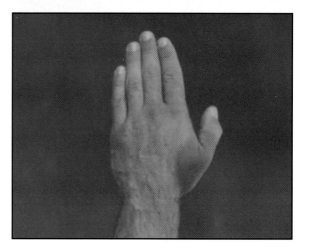

ORIGIN

Lateral border of the third metacarpal.

INSERTION

Base of the proximal phalanx.

RPP

Radial and palmar aspects of the thumb.

TP

Web space. Pincer palpation from the palmar and volar surfaces.

MFS

Thumb abduction; you may try both palmar and radial abduction.

PSS

Pain at the first metacarpophalangeal joint.

HEP

As MFS above with the patient using the other thumb and fingers to facilitate stretch.

BIOMECHANICS OF INJURY

See abductor pollicis brevis.

CLINICAL NOTES

All thenar muscles may participate in a "trigger thumb" condition. Make sure the palpation is on the adductor pollicis and <u>not</u> on the first dorsal interosseous.

TRIGGER POINT THERAPY

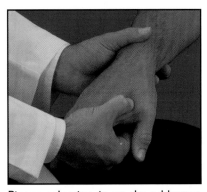

Pincer palpation is on the adductor pollicis and <u>not</u> on the first dorsal interosseous.

MYOFASCIAL STRETCHES

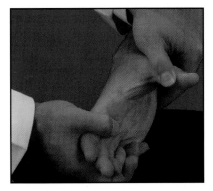

HOME EXERCISE PROGRAM

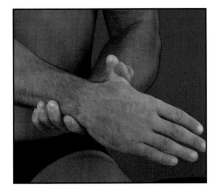

OPPONENS POLLICIS

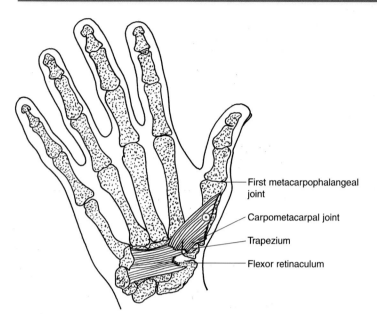

First metacarpophalangeal joint

Carpometacarpal joint

Trapezium

Flexor retinaculum

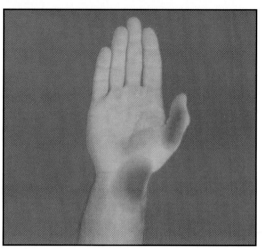

ORIGIN

Tubercle of the trapezium and flexor retinaculum.

INSERTION

First metacarpal.

RPP

Areas of origin and insertion of the muscle.

TP

Midpoint of a line drawn between the radial aspect of the carpometacarpal and MP-1 joints.

MFS

Same as flexor pollicis brevis.

PSS

Pain at the first metacarpophalangeal joint.

HEP

As MFS above with the patient using the other thumb and fingers to facilitate stretch.

BIOMECHANICS OF INJURY

See abductor pollicis brevis.

CLINICAL NOTES

All thenar muscles may participate in a "trigger thumb" condition.

TRIGGER POINT THERAPY

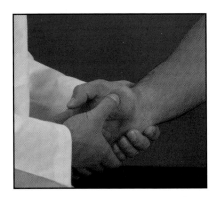

MYOFASCIAL STRETCHES

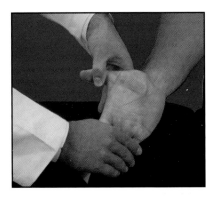

HOME EXERCISE PROGRAM

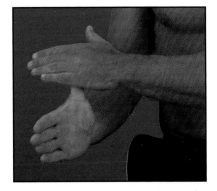

ABDOMINAL REGION

RECTUS ABDOMINIS

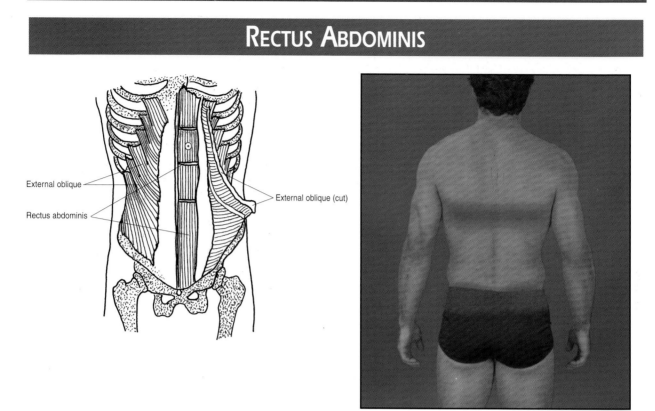

External oblique

Rectus abdominis

External oblique (cut)

ORIGIN

Pubic crest and the ligament in front of the pubic symphysis.

INSERTION

Xiphoid process and over the costal margin of the seventh to fifth cartilages.

RPP

Across the lumbar and midthoracic spine.

TP

Inferior and lateral to the xiphoid process.

MFS

Extension of the trunk using a therapeutic exercise ball while the clinician facilitates stretching.

PSS

Low back pain.

HEP

The patient applies a similar stretch using a table or therapeutic exercise ball.

BIOMECHANICS OF INJURY

Acute overload, lifting heavy objects, stress, poor posture.

CLINICAL NOTES

Proceed with care when facilitating trunk extension so as not to injure the lumbar spine.

TRIGGER POINT THERAPY

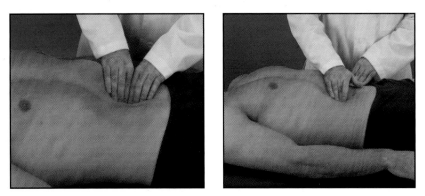

MYOFASCIAL STRETCHES

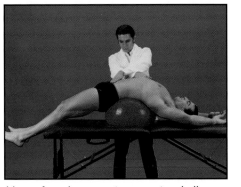

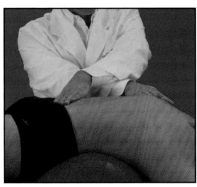

Use of a therapeutic exercise ball can facilitate stretching of the rectus abdominis muscle.

HOME EXERCISE PROGRAM

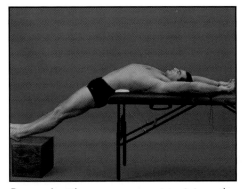

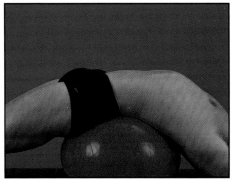

Proceed with care so as not to injure the lumbar spine.

DIAPHRAGM

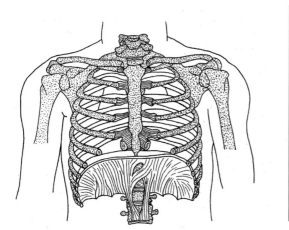
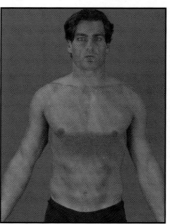
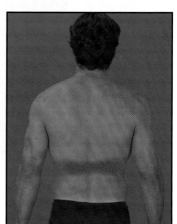

ORIGIN

Its musculature is peripheral and radiates from the sternum to the ribs to the costal cartilages, and from the lumbar vertebrae toward the central tendon.

INSERTION

Lower thoracic to upper lumbar vertebrae.

RPP

Chest pain, dyspnea, inability to get a full breath, and low back pain.

TP

Under the rib cage. The clinician stands behind the patient and uses all fingers to apply trigger point therapy. Facilitate pressure during exhalation.

MFS

Inhaling deeply with relaxed abdominal muscles.

PSS

None detected.

HEP

Complete exhalation followed by a full inhalation while relaxing the abdominal muscles.

BIOMECHANICS OF INJURY

Prolonged shallow breathing, constant coughing.

TRIGGER POINT THERAPY

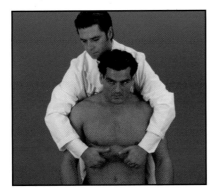

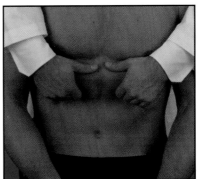

As the patient exhales, the clinician facilitates a progressive pressure technique on the trigger point region.

MYOFASCIAL STRETCHES AND HOME EXERCISE PROGRAM

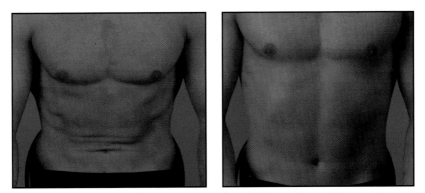

Complete exhalation followed by complete full inhalation while relaxing the abdominal muscles.

THORACOLUMBAR SPINE REGION

RHOMBOIDEUS MAJOR

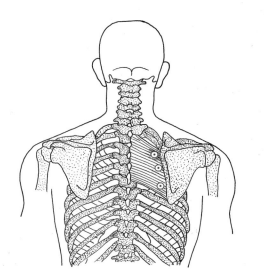

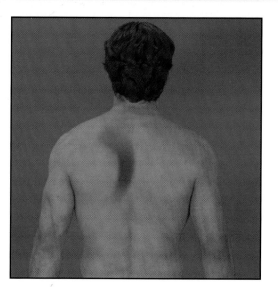

ORIGIN

Spinous processes of T2 to T5.

INSERTION

Vertebral border of the scapula.

RPP

Along the medial border of the scapula.

TP

Various trigger points can be identified two FBs medial to the vertebral border of the scapula. Use flat palpation.

MFS

The patient is in a sitting position with the neck flexed and arms crossed. The patient moves into forward flexion, spreading the crossed arms over the legs. The clinician facilitates scapular abduction.

PSS

None detected.

HEP

The patient flexes the arms forward to 90 degrees and pulls the body backward, reinforcing scapular abduction.

BIOMECHANICS OF INJURY

Weight lifting from a prone position for rhomboids strengthening. Working for long hours in a forward leaned position with arms in forward extended flexion that causes scapular abduction. Upper crossed syndrome may cause myofascial trigger points via prolonged overstretching of the rhomboids.

TRIGGER POINT THERAPY

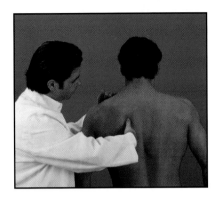

MYOFASCIAL STRETCHES

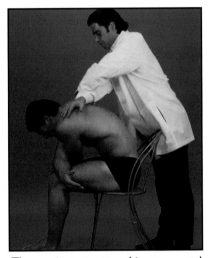   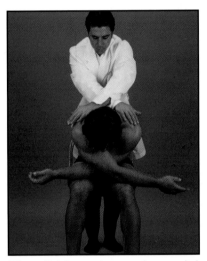

The patient crosses his arms and facilitates scapular abduction.

The clinician palpates the medial border of both scapulae and spreads them apart to create scapular abduction.

HOME EXERCISE PROGRAM

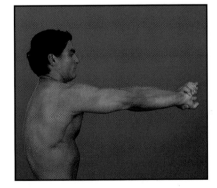

MIDDLE AND LOWER TRAPEZIUS

First cervical vertebra

Seventh cervical vertebra

Spine of scapula

Inferior angle of scapula

Trapezius
(upper)
(middle)
(lower)

Twelfth
thoracic
vertebra

Middle Trapezius   **Lower Trapezius**

ORIGIN

Middle—C7 and upper thoracic vertebrae.
Lower—Lower thoracic vertebrae.

INSERTION

Middle—Acromion process and spine of the scapula.
Lower—Spine of the scapula.

RPP

Posterolateral aspect of the neck; suprascapular and interscapular regions.

TP

Middle—Midway between the midpoint of the spine of the scapula and the spinous process of the vertebra at the same level.
Lower—On a line perpendicular to the vertebral column at the level of the inferior angle of the scapula, two FB from the spinous process of that vertebra.

MFS

Middle—The patient is seated with neck flexion and crossed arms, reinforcing scapular abduction. The clinician facilitates stretch.
Lower—The patient is seated with neck and trunk flexion and arms flexed forward. The clinician facilitates stretch.

PSS

None detected.

HEP

Same as MFS.

BIOMECHANICS OF INJURY

Activities or positions that include prolonged overstretching or overshortening of the muscle by maintaining arms in a forward flexed position. Active overlengthening of the muscle when driving a car and holding onto a steering wheel with both hands for a prolonged time.

CLINICAL NOTES

Upper crossed syndrome with tight pectoralis muscles may cause activation of the middle trapezius through prolonged overstretching.

TRIGGER POINT THERAPY

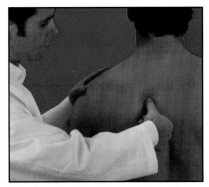

The myofascial trigger point of the middle trapezius muscle.

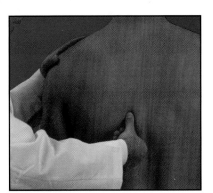

The myofascial trigger point of the lower trapezius muscle.

MYOFASCIAL STRETCHES

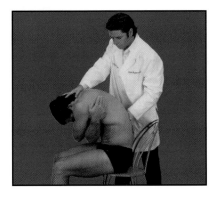

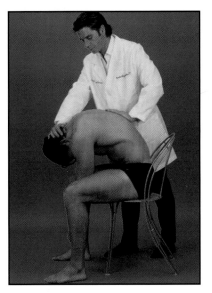

HOME EXERCISE PROGRAM

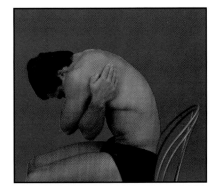

ILIOCOSTALIS THORACIS

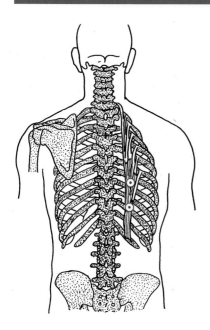
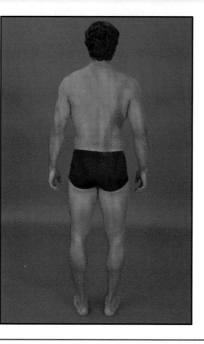
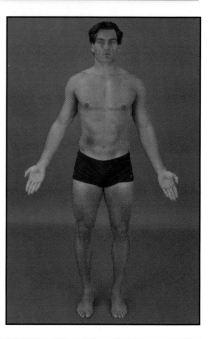

ORIGIN

Inferior six ribs.

INSERTION

Angles of the superior six ribs.

RPP

Along the muscle belly, inferior angle of the scapula, and superior abdominal area of the same side.

TP

Along the belly of the muscle. Flat palpation.

MFS

The patient is in a long sitting position. He or she flexes the trunk forward and reaches with the arm to the opposite side. The clinician facilitates stretching of the muscle.

PSS

Not detected.

HEP

The patient is in a sitting position and leaning forward, stretching the muscle.

BIOMECHANICS OF INJURY

Scoliosis, kyphosis, leg length discrepancy, sudden twisting or bending.

CLINICAL NOTES

The referred pain to the superior abdominal area is rather frequent, and differential diagnosis between myofascial trigger point syndrome and visceral involvement must be clear.

TRIGGER POINT THERAPY

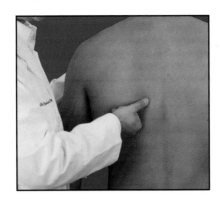

MYOFASCIAL STRETCHES

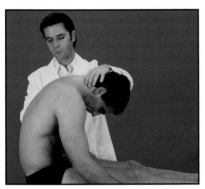 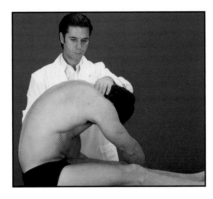 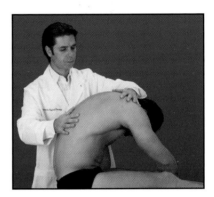

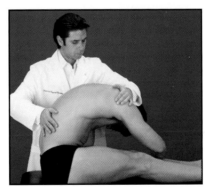

HOME EXERCISE PROGRAM

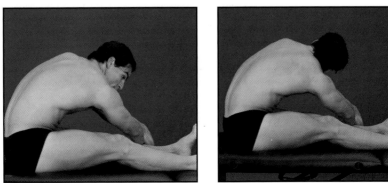

ILIOCOSTALIS LUMBORUM

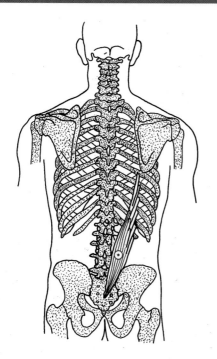
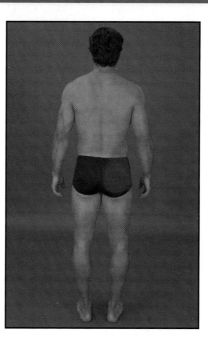

ORIGIN

Iliac crest.

INSERTION

Angles of the inferior six or seven ribs.

RPP

Along the muscle belly and buttock area.

TP

Along the muscle belly. Flat palpation.

MFS

The patient is in a long sitting position and flexes the trunk forward, reaching with the arm to the opposite side. The clinician facilitates stretching of the muscle.

PSS

Not detected.

HEP

The patient is in a sitting position and leaning forward, stretching the muscle.

BIOMECHANICS OF INJURY

Scoliosis, kyphosis, leg length discrepancy, sudden twisting or bending.

TRIGGER POINT THERAPY

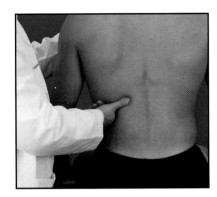

MYOFASCIAL STRETCHES

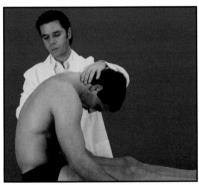 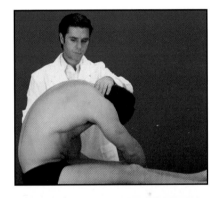 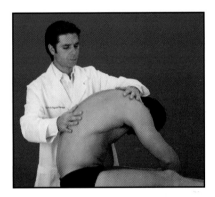

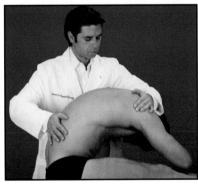

HOME EXERCISE PROGRAM

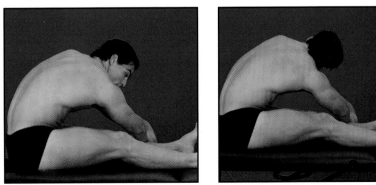

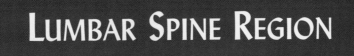

LUMBAR SPINE REGION

QUADRATUS LUMBORUM

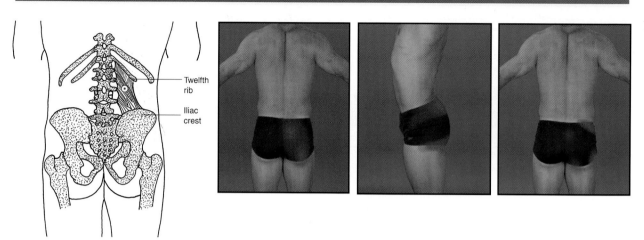

ORIGIN

Iliolumbar ligament, adjacent part of the iliac crest, and inferior two to four lumbar transverse processes.

INSERTION

Twelfth rib, tips of the transverse processes of L1 to L4 vertebrae.

RPP

Sacroiliac joint, lower buttock, belly of the muscle.

TP

Several trigger points—three FB lateral to the transverse processes of L1 to L4. Deep, flat palpation.

MFS

Position 1—The patient is in a semiprone position with the leg in extension and adduction. The clinician supports the area of the lower thoracic cage and iliac crest with his hands while spreading the hands apart.
Position 2—The patient is in a semisupine position with the leg in flexion and adduction. The clinician supports the area of the lower thoracic cage and iliac crest with his hands while spreading the hands apart.

PSS

Pain at the contralateral lumbar spine.

HEP

The patient is in a standing position and side-bends to the opposite side. Slight flexion may further facilitate the stretch.

BIOMECHANICS OF INJURY

Lifting objects from the floor, awkward torso movements, loss of balance during a movement, bending and twisting the trunk for a prolonged time or repetitively, leg length discrepancies, scoliosis.

CLINICAL NOTES

During trigger point therapy and while the patient is in a sidelying position, place the patient's arm in extension to elevate the rib cage; leg is in extension and adduction to drop the iliac crest lower, and use a pillow or bolster under the nontreated side to open up a wider space where trigger points can be easier identified.

TRIGGER POINT THERAPY

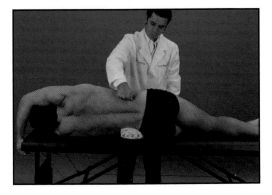
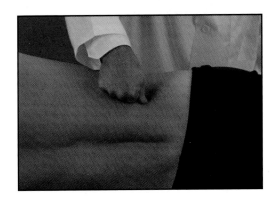

MYOFASCIAL STRETCHES

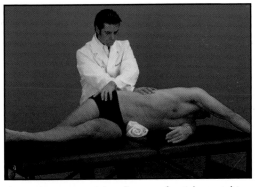
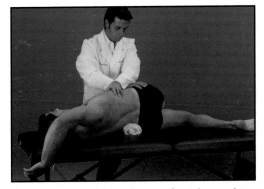

A semiprone position for myofascial stretching
of the quadratus lumborum.

A semisupine position for myofascial stretching
of the quadratus lumborum.

HOME EXERCISE PROGRAM

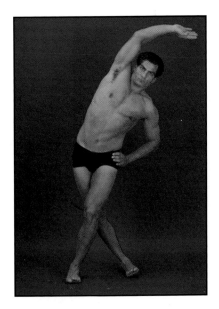

ILIOPSOAS

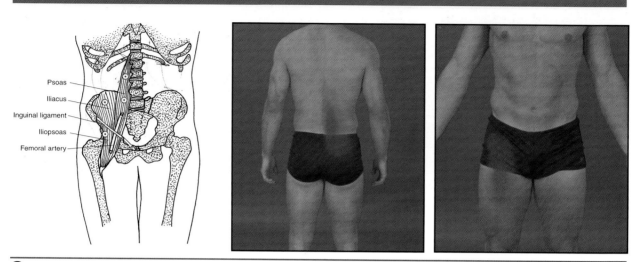

ORIGIN

Psoas major, T12 to L5 vertebrae and intervertebral discs. Iliacus, iliac crest, fossa and ala of the sacrum.

INSERTION

Lesser trochanter of the femur.

RPP

Low back, anterior and anteromedial thigh, buttock area, sacroiliac joint.

TP

Iliopsoas—Two FB lateral to the femoral artery and one FB below the inguinal ligament. Flat palpation with the thumb. Iliacus—Anterior to the inner surface of the iliac crest, immediately cephalad to the anterior superior iliac spine (ASIS). Flat palpation ("hook style") with four fingers.
Psoas major intra-abdominal point—Midline between the ASIS and midline of the body. Use flat palpation with both hands and aim in a posteromedial direction. Ask the patient to flex the hip to confirm correct location.

MFS

Position 1: The patient is in supine position. The involved leg is suspended off the table while the uninvolved leg with knee flexed stabilizes the pelvis. The clinician gently facilitates hip extension. Position 2: The patient is in a half-kneeling position. The knee of the involved side is on a pillow. The arm is flexed to 180 degrees. The clinician is standing behind the patient and assists forward movement in order to facilitate further stretch of the iliopsoas by extending the hip and slightly extending the lumbar spine.

PSS

Pain at the lumbar spine area.

HEP

1. Standing stretch: The patient is in standing position. Note that the majority of the extension action is from the hip and not from the lumbar spine. 2. Kneeling stretch: The patient is in a half-kneeling position, described in MFS.

BIOMECHANICS OF INJURY

High-velocity injuries during falls or sports injuries. Acute overshortening of the muscle in extreme sitting positions. Repetitive movements of hip flexion, as in driving for long hours and using the hip flexors for using the car pedals. Lumbar disc herniation, scoliosis, and lumbar fusion may activate trigger points in the muscle.

CLINICAL NOTES

The iliopsoas may entrap the genitofemoral nerve, causing paresthesias at the scrotal and labial areas. It may also participate in entrapment of the lateral femoral cutaneous nerve, causing meralgia paresthetica.

TRIGGER POINT THERAPY

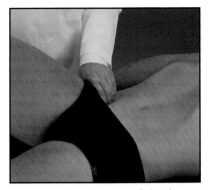

Trigger point palpation of the iliacus muscle.

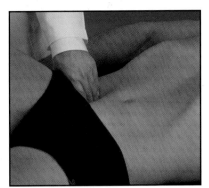

Intra-abdominal trigger point palpation of the psoas major muscle.

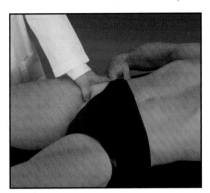

Common iliopsoas muscle trigger point palpation.

MYOFASCIAL STRETCHES

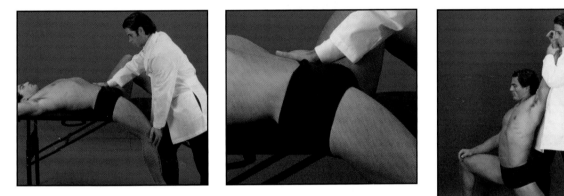

HOME EXERCISE PROGRAM

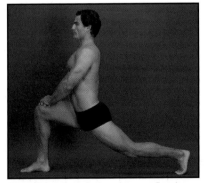

Standing stretch involves a flat lumbar spine. The knee of the stretched side must be extended to facilitate further hip extension.

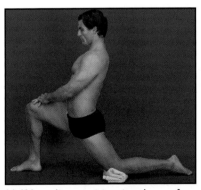

Half-kneeling position involves a forward movement of the pelvis, stretching the iliopsoas muscles.

Gluteus Maximus

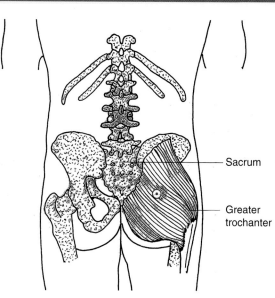

Sacrum

Greater trochanter

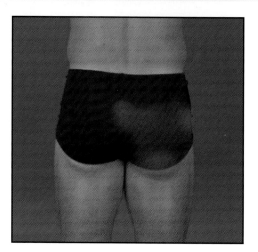

Origin

Posterior surface of the sacrum and iliac crest.

Insertion

Iliotibial tract and linea aspera of the femur.

RPP

Buttock area and sacrum.

TP

Midway between the greater trochanter and the sacrum. Flat palpation.

MFS

Hip flexion. The clinician facilitates movement.

PSS

Pain in the groin area.

HEP

The patient is in a supine position and brings the hip into flexion, facilitating movement with both hands.

Biomechanics of Injury

Sports injuries and falls may activate trigger points.

Clinical Notes

See the gluteus medius.

TRIGGER POINT THERAPY

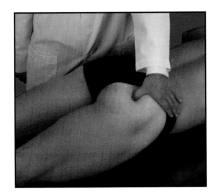

MYOFASCIAL STRETCHES

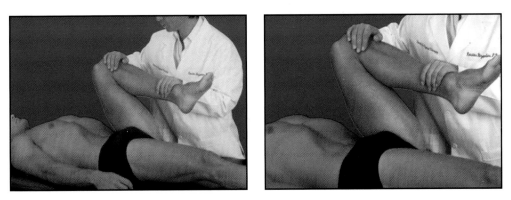

HOME EXERCISE PROGRAM

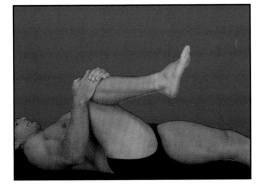

GLUTEUS MEDIUS

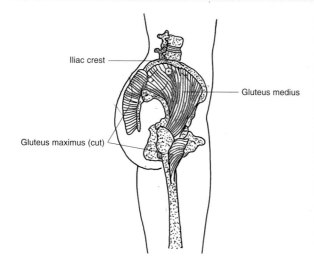

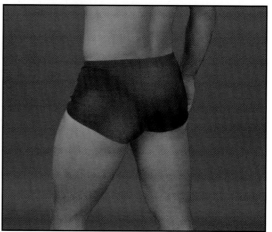

ORIGIN

Outer surface of the iliac crest.

INSERTION

Greater trochanter of the femur.

RPP

Low back, posterior crest of the ilium, sacrum, and buttock.

TP

Two FB below the midpoint of the outer surface of iliac crest. Flat palpation.

MFS

Hip flexion and adduction. The clinician facilitates movement.

PSS

Pain in the groin area.

HEP

The patient is in a supine position. The involved side is in hip flexion and adduction. The patient facilitates movement using one hand to assist hip flexion and the other to assist hip adduction.

BIOMECHANICS OF INJURY

Sudden falls and sports injuries.

CLINICAL NOTES

A Morton's foot condition may perpetuate myofascial trigger points in the muscle. In a Morton's foot condition, the first metatarsal is short while the second is longer and drops lower than the first. Consequently, in the "push-off" phase of gait, the second metatarsal will contact the ground first and weightbearing will push the foot into pronation. Pronation will further cause tibial rotation and the appearance of a genu valgum with femoral medial rotation and adduction. The gluteus medius will be exposed to repetitive overstretching. This will cause perpetuation of trigger points. The condition can be corrected by orthotics.

TRIGGER POINT THERAPY

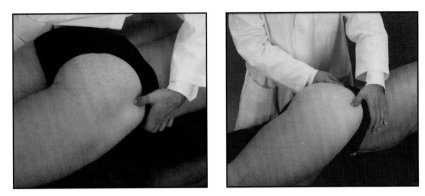

MYOFASCIAL STRETCHES

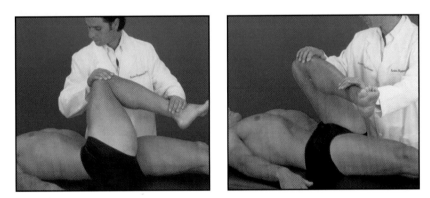

HOME EXERCISE PROGRAM

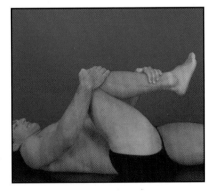

GLUTEUS MINIMUS

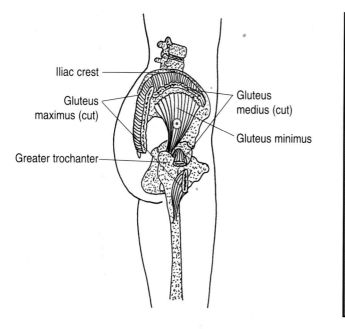

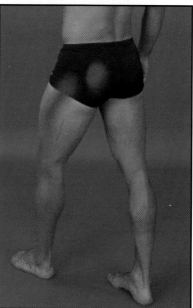

ORIGIN

Outer surface of the ilium, between the anterior and inferior gluteal lines.

INSERTION

Anterior surface of the greater trochanter of the femur.

RPP

Belly of the muscle, lateral aspect of the thigh, knee, leg and ankle, posterior thigh, and calf.

TP

Midway between the midpoint of the iliac crest and greater trochanter of the femur. Flat palpation through the fibers of gluteus medius.

MFS

Hip flexion, adduction, and external rotation. The clinician facilitates movement.

PSS

Not detected.

HEP

The patient is in a supine position. The involved side is in hip flexion, adduction, and external rotation. The patient facilitates movement using one hand to assist hip flexion and adduction and the other to assist external rotation.

BIOMECHANICS OF INJURY

Sports injuries, falls, attempting to prevent an object from falling down.

TRIGGER POINT THERAPY

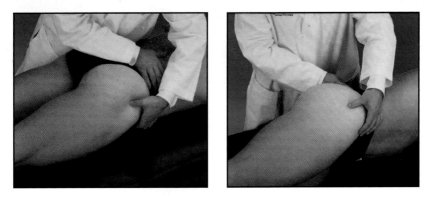

MYOFASCIAL STRETCHES

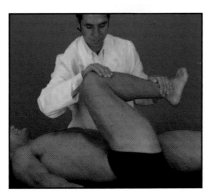

HOME EXERCISE PROGRAM

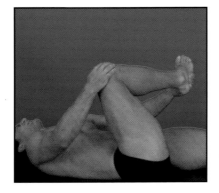

PIRIFORMIS

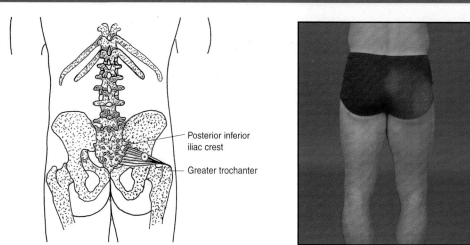

Posterior inferior
iliac crest

Greater trochanter

ORIGIN

Anterior surface of the sacrum.

INSERTION

Superior border of the greater trochanter.

RPP

Sacroiliac region, lateral buttock region, and posterior thigh.

TP

Midpoint between the posterior inferior iliac spine and the greater trochanter. Flat palpation using the thumb or fingers of both hands moving through the fibers of the gluteus maximus, reaching the piriformis muscle.

MFS

Hip flexion (above 90 degrees), adduction, and external rotation with emphasis on external rotation. The clinician facilitates movements in the above-mentioned order.

PSS

Not detected.

HEP

The patient is in a supine position. The involved side is in hip flexion above 90 degrees, adduction, and external rotation. Emphasis is on external rotation. The patient facilitates movement using one hand to assist hip flexion and adduction and the other to assist external rotation.

BIOMECHANICS OF INJURY

Acute overload through sudden movements or picking up and lifting objects, prolonged periods of driving or sitting, sports injuries.

CLINICAL NOTES

In a small percentage of the population (less than 1%), both the tibial and peroneal divisions of the sciatic nerve penetrate and pass through the fibers of the piriformis muscle (anatomical variation). Piriformis syndrome may occur when acute spasm of the piriformis is present in those patients with this anatomical variation. Differential diagnosis between a true piriformis syndrome and a piriformis myofascial trigger point involvement is necessary.

TRIGGER POINT THERAPY

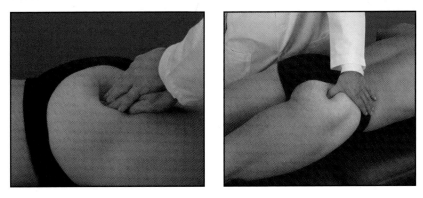

MYOFASCIAL STRETCHES

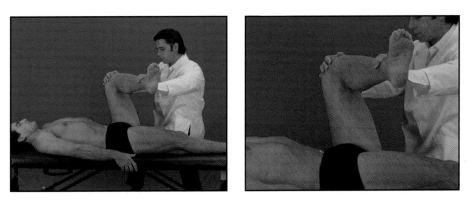

HOME EXERCISE PROGRAM

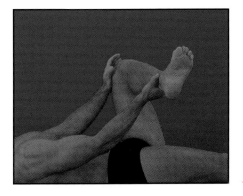

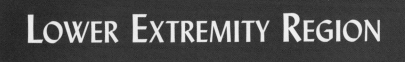

LOWER EXTREMITY REGION

ADDUCTOR MAGNUS

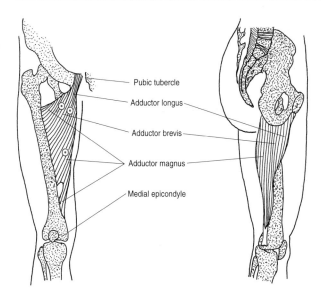

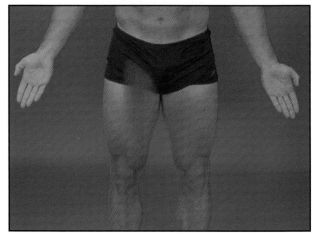

Pubic tubercle
Adductor longus
Adductor brevis
Adductor magnus
Medial epicondyle

ORIGIN

Inferior ramus of the pubis, ramus of the ischium, and the ischial tuberosity.

INSERTION

Gluteal tuberosity, linea aspera, and adductor tubercle of the femur.

RPP

Anterior and medial aspects of the thigh up to the knee.

TP

In the midline between the pubic tubercle and the medial epicondyle of the femur. Pincer or flat palpation can be used.

MFS

Hip abduction and external rotation.

PSS

Not detected.

HEP

The patient is in supine position and slides the foot of the involved side in the inner surface of the leg of the uninvolved side. The resulting action is abduction and external rotation.

BIOMECHANICS OF INJURY

Myofascial dysfunction of the iliopsoas muscle may activate satellite trigger points in the adductor magnus.

CLINICAL NOTES

In cases of lumbar spine pathology when the iliopsoas is myofascially involved, low back and anterior thigh pain may exist. Treatment of the iliopsoas muscle will resolve both areas of pain in most cases. Occasionally, though, the anterior thigh pain may remain until treatment of the adductor magnus takes place.

TRIGGER POINT THERAPY

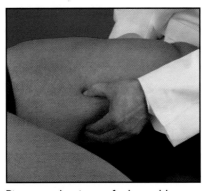 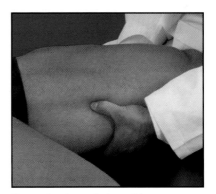

Pincer palpation of the adductor magnus trigger point.

Flat palpation of the adductor magnus trigger point.

MYOFASCIAL STRETCHES

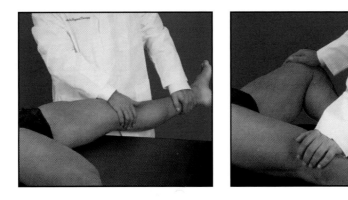

HOME EXERCISE PROGRAM

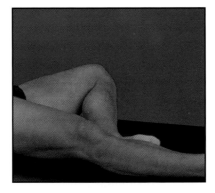

PECTINEUS

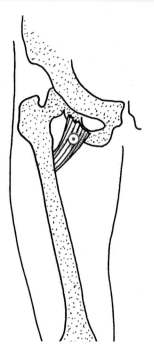 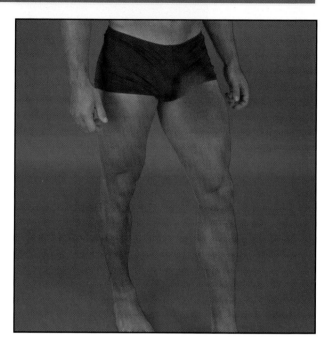

ORIGIN

Superior ramus of the pubis.

INSERTION

Below the lesser trochanter of the femur.

RPP

Groin area and upper anteromedial thigh.

TP

One FB lateral to the pubic tubercle with flat palpation.

MFS

The patient is in a supine position. The clinician facilitates abduction and extension of the hip.

PSS

Not detected.

HEP

The patient is in a sitting position and brings the involved leg into knee flexion, hip extension, and abduction. From a standing position, the patient facilitates hip abduction with some extension. The patient uses the hand to gently push the hip anteriorly and facilitate movement.

BIOMECHANICS OF INJURY

Sudden falls, sports activities, riding a motorcycle, horseback riding.

TRIGGER POINT THERAPY

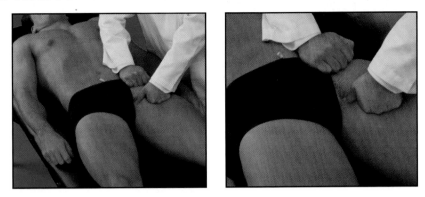

MYOFASCIAL STRETCHES

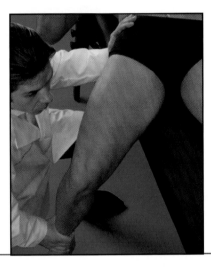

HOME EXERCISE PROGRAM

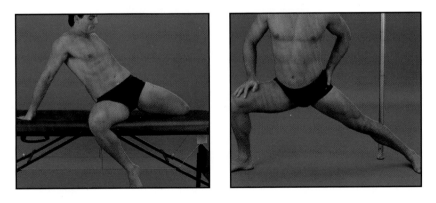

TENSOR FASCIAE LATAE

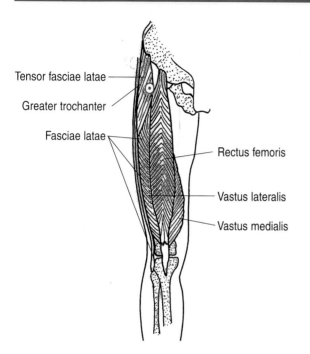

Tensor fasciae latae
Greater trochanter
Fasciae latae
Rectus femoris
Vastus lateralis
Vastus medialis

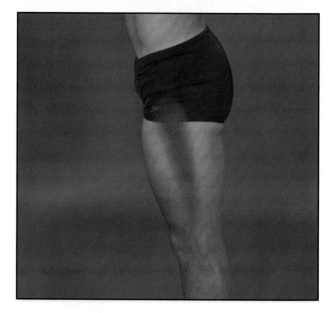

ORIGIN

Anterior superior iliac spine and external lip of the iliac crest.

INSERTION

The tensor fasciae latae tendon inserts into the lateral condyle of the tibia.

RPP

Anterior and lateral aspects of the thigh, extending to the knee area.

TP

Three FB anterior to the greater trochanter of the femur. Use flat palpation with the thumb.

MFS

The patient is in a sidelying position with hip extension and adduction while the clinician facilitates movement and stabilizes the pelvis.

PSS

Not detected.

HEP

The patient is in a standing position; the hip of the involved side is in extension and adduction. The patient shifts the body lateral and anterior toward the involved side.

BIOMECHANICS OF INJURY

Sports injuries, especially in marathon runners. Overshortening of the muscle may occur in cases of prolonged immobilization.

TRIGGER POINT THERAPY

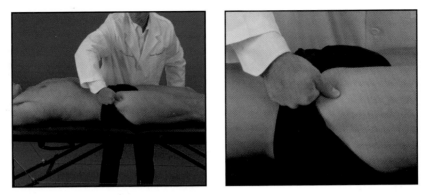

MYOFASCIAL STRETCHES

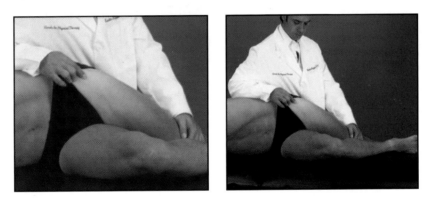

HOME EXERCISE PROGRAM

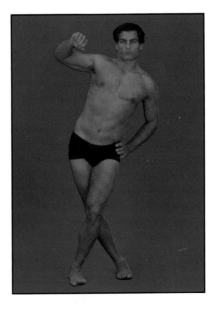

RECTUS FEMORIS

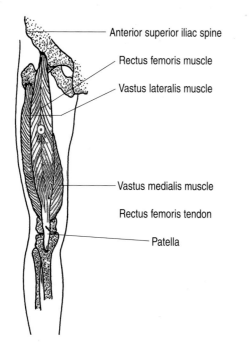

- Anterior superior iliac spine
- Rectus femoris muscle
- Vastus lateralis muscle
- Vastus medialis muscle
- Rectus femoris tendon
- Patella

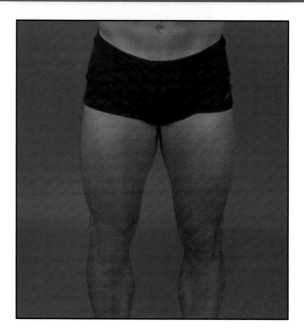

ORIGIN

Anterior inferior iliac spin.

INSERTION

Base of the patella and through the quadriceps tendon to the tibial tuberosity.

RPP

Anterior thigh area; suprapatellar pain.

TP

Midway between the anterior superior iliac spine (ASIS) and the superior border of patella. Use flat palpation.

MFS

Knee flexion with the hip neutral or in extension. The patient can be in a supine, prone, or sidelying position.

PSS

Deep knee pain.

HEP

The patient is in a standing position and holds the leg from the foot and facilitates knee flexion and hip extension.

BIOMECHANICS OF INJURY

Myofascial dysfunction of the iliopsoas muscle may activate satellite trigger points in the rectus femoris.

CLINICAL NOTES

Combined tightness of the iliopsoas and rectus femoris may cause limitation in knee flexion.

TRIGGER POINT THERAPY

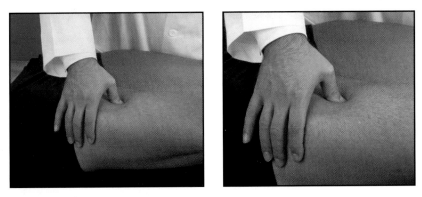

MYOFASCIAL STRETCHES

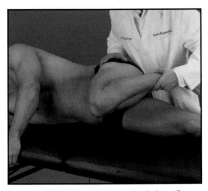

The patient is sidelying with hip flexion. The clinician takes up the slack of the muscle and facilitates complete knee flexion.

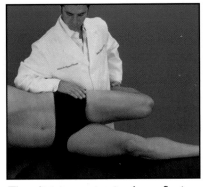

The clinician maintains knee flexion and brings the hip into extension.

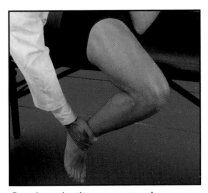

Combined iliopsoas and rectus femoris stretch from the supine position. The clinician facilitates knee flexion.

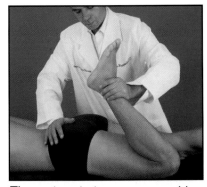

The patient is in a prone position and the clinician facilitates stretch.

HOME EXERCISE PROGRAM

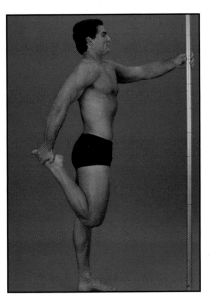

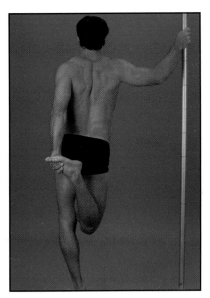

Vastus Medialis

Anterior superior iliac spine

Rectus femoris muscle

Vastus lateralis muscle

Vastus intermedius muscle

Vastus medialis muscle

Rectus femoris tendon

Patella

ORIGIN

Medial linea aspera and intertrochanteric line.

INSERTION

Base of the patella and through the quadriceps tendon to the tibial tuberosity.

RPP

Medial aspect of the knee and thigh.

TP

Four FB above the medial superior border of the patella. Use flat palpation.

MFS

Same as the rectus femoris.

PSS

Deep knee pain.

HEP

The patient is in a standing position and holds the leg from the foot and facilitates knee flexion and hip extension. Use the hand of the same side to stretch.

BIOMECHANICS OF INJURY

Arthritic conditions, knee arthroscopies, and other surgical interventions of the knee may cause activation of trigger points.

TRIGGER POINT THERAPY

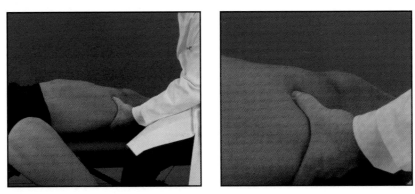

MYOFASCIAL STRETCHES

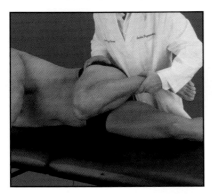
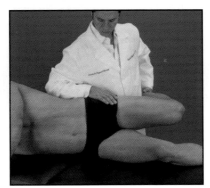
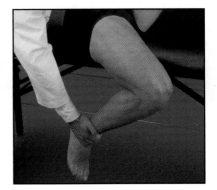

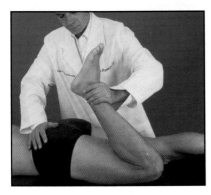

HOME EXERCISE PROGRAM

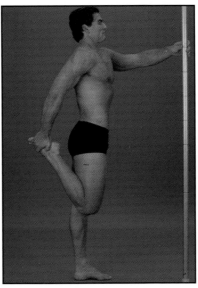
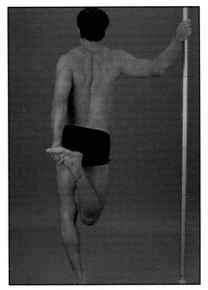

Vastus Medialis   **Vastus Lateralis**

VASTUS LATERALIS

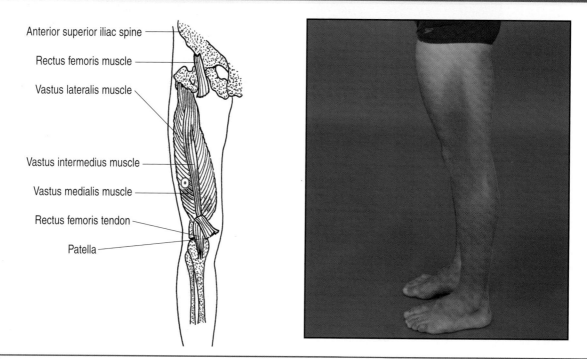

Anterior superior iliac spine
Rectus femoris muscle
Vastus lateralis muscle
Vastus intermedius muscle
Vastus medialis muscle
Rectus femoris tendon
Patella

ORIGIN

Greater trochanter and lateral linea aspera of the femur.

INSERTION

Base of the patella and through the quadriceps tendon to the tibial tuberosity.

RPP

Lateral knee and lateral thigh pain.

TP

One HB above the lateral superior border of the patella.

MFS

Same as the rectus femoris.

PSS

Deep knee pain.

HEP

The patient is in a standing position and holds the leg from the foot and facilitates knee flexion and hip extension. Use the contralateral hand.

BIOMECHANICS OF INJURY

Sports accidents as in skiing; immobilization of the knee joint.

CLINICAL NOTES

A common pitfall into which clinicians can fall is to palpate the iliotibial band instead of the vastus lateralis muscle.

TRIGGER POINT THERAPY

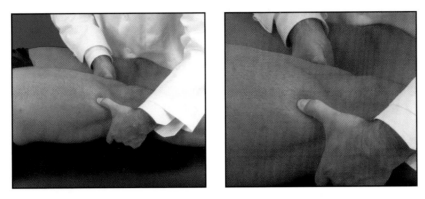

MYOFASCIAL STRETCHES

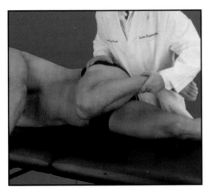
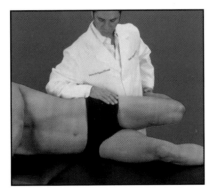
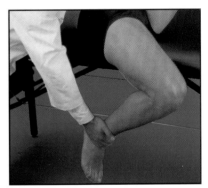

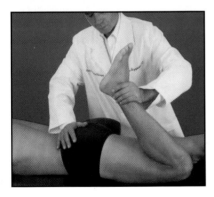

HOME EXERCISE PROGRAM

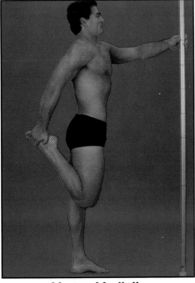
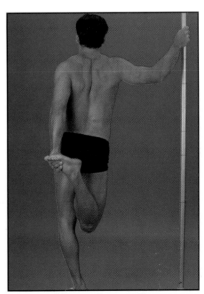

Vastus Medialis   **Vastus Lateralis**

VASTUS INTERMEDIUS

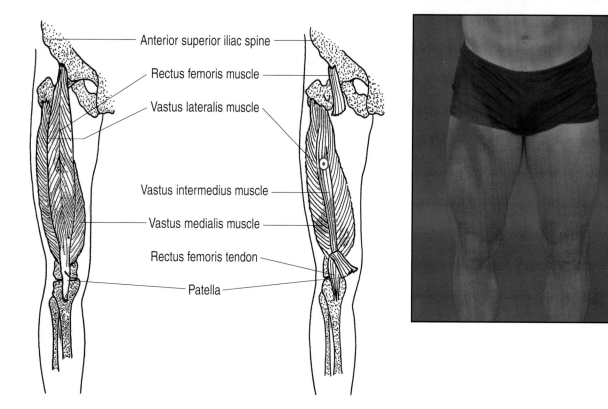

Anterior superior iliac spine

Rectus femoris muscle

Vastus lateralis muscle

Vastus intermedius muscle

Vastus medialis muscle

Rectus femoris tendon

Patella

ORIGIN

Anterolateral surface of the body of the femur.

INSERTION

Base of the patella and through the quadriceps tendon to the tibial tuberosity.

RPP

Anterior thigh.

TP

Midway between the ASIS and superior border of the patella, under the trigger point of the rectus femoris.

MFS

Same as the rectus femoris.

PSS

Deep knee pain.

HEP

The patient is in a standing position and holds the leg from the foot and facilitates knee flexion and hip extension.

BIOMECHANICS OF INJURY

Myofascial dysfunction of the rectus femoris muscle may activate satellite trigger points in the vastus intermedius.

TRIGGER POINT THERAPY

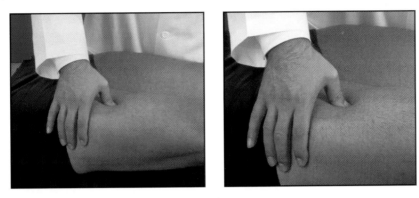

MYOFASCIAL STRETCHES

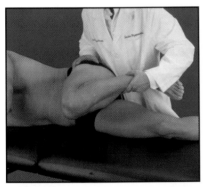
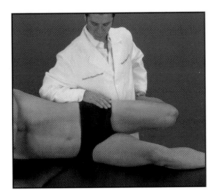
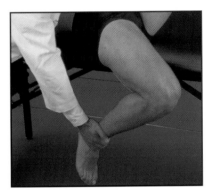

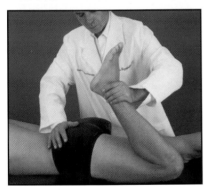

HOME EXERCISE PROGRAM

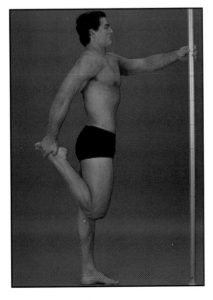
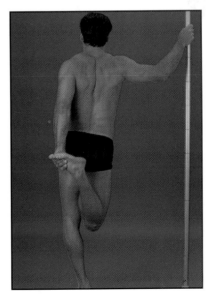

BICEPS FEMORIS (LONG AND SHORT HEADS)

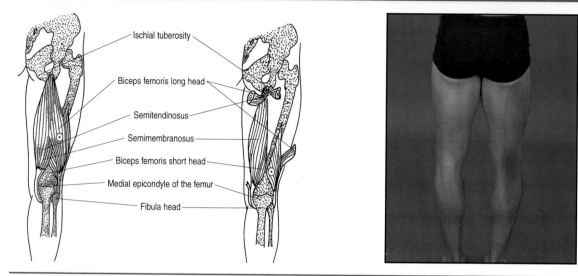

ORIGIN

Biceps femoris long head—Ischial tuberosity.
Biceps femoris short head—Linea aspera and lateral supracondylar line.

INSERTION

Biceps femoris—Fibular head.

RPP

Posterior and lateral aspects of the thigh; posterior aspect of knee.

TP

Biceps femoris long head—Midpoint between the ischial tuberosity and the fibular head.
Biceps femoris short head—Four FB above the fibular head, medial to the tendon of the biceps femoris long head.

MFS

The patient is in a supine position and the knee is extended. The clinician facilitates stretching from hip flexion-abduction-external rotation to hip flexion-adduction-internal rotation.

PSS

Low back and deep knee pain.

HEP

The patient is in a standing position and flexes the hip of the involved side with the leg resting on a table and the knee extended. The patient leans with the body, anteriorly facilitating stretch.

BIOMECHANICS OF INJURY

Direct trauma, usually in sports injuries. Prolonged sitting or bedrest can cause activation of trigger points through over-shortening.

CLINICAL NOTES

Myofascial involvement of the hamstrings and gastrocnemius muscle may cause limitation of knee extension greater than 7 degrees.

TRIGGER POINT THERAPY

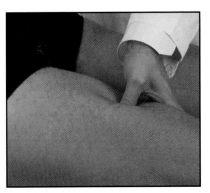 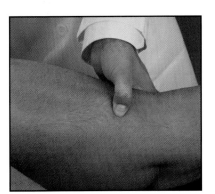

Semitendinosus trigger point.   Semimembranosus muscle.

MYOFASCIAL STRETCHES

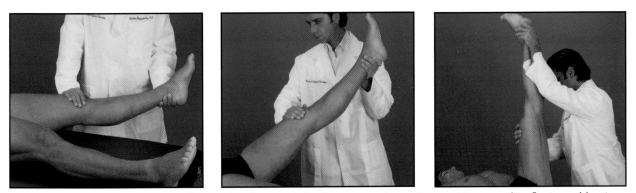

The clinician facilitates stretching from a hip flexion-abduction-external rotation position to a hip flexion-adduction-internal rotation position in order to achieve a complete stretch,

HOME EXERCISE PROGRAM

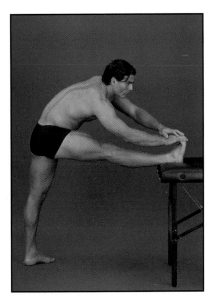

POPLITEUS

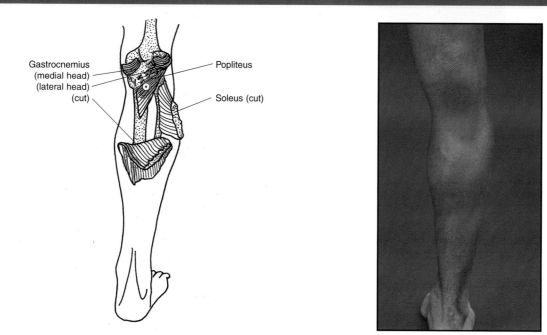

Gastrocnemius
(medial head)
(lateral head)
(cut)

Popliteus

Soleus (cut)

ORIGIN

Lateral condyle of the femur.

INSERTION

Posterior tibia.

RPP

Entire knee area with emphasis on the posterior aspect of the knee.

TP

Two FB below and one FB medial to the midline crossing the popliteal crease, directly on the posterior surface of the tibia. Flat palpation. The patient can be placed in a prone or supine position.

MFS

The patient is in a long sitting position with the knee fully extended. The clinician facilitates ankle dorsiflexion that causes tibial rotation.

PSS

Deep knee pain.

HEP

Same as MFS above. The patient uses a towel to assist in stretching.

BIOMECHANICS OF INJURY

Knee immobilization, surgical interventions, sports injuries.

CLINICAL NOTES

Myofascial involvement of the popliteus muscle may cause limitation of knee extension less than 7 degrees.

TRIGGER POINT THERAPY

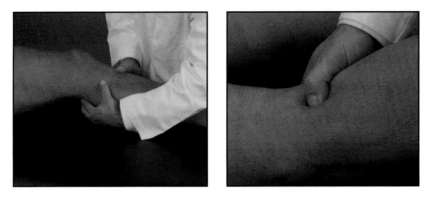

MYOFASCIAL STRETCHES

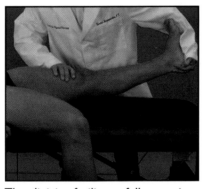

The clinician facilitates full extension
of the knee and ankle dorsiflexion.

HOME EXERCISE PROGRAM

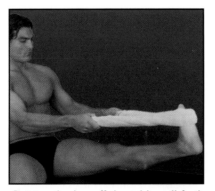
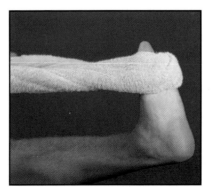

Raising the leg off the table will facilitate greater knee hyperextension.

GASTROCNEMIUS

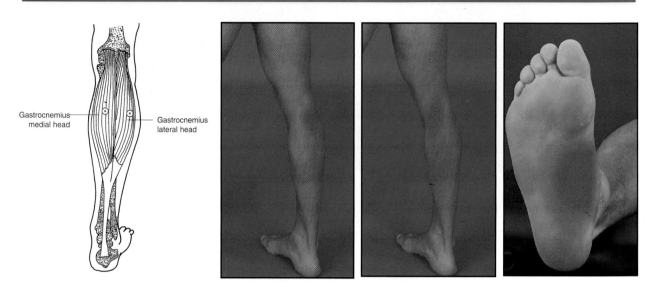

Gastrocnemius medial head — Gastrocnemius lateral head

ORIGIN

Lateral head—Lateral femoral condyle.
Medial head—Medial femoral condyle.

INSERTION

Posterior knee, lower third of the posterior thigh, along the belly of the muscle, Achilles' tendon area, ankle and foot.

RPP

Belly of the muscle, Achilles' tendon, sole of the foot.

TP

Lateral head—One HB below the lateral aspect of the popliteal crease.
Medial head—One HB below the medial aspect of the popliteal crease.

MFS

The clinician facilitates dorsiflexion of the ankle with the knee completely extended.

PSS

Pain at the anterior ankle area.

HEP

The patient is in a standing position and stretches against the wall. He positions the foot to be stretched behind the other foot and leans anteriorly, causing ankle dorsiflexion with the knee extended.

BIOMECHANICS OF INJURY

Climbing uphill, immobilization after ankle fractures.

CLINICAL NOTES

In cases of Achilles' tendonitis, the gastrocnemius should be treated together with the soleus and tibialis posterior muscles. The gastrocnemius can be myofascially involved and, thus, appropriate to be treated in cases of plantarfasciitis.

ERAPY

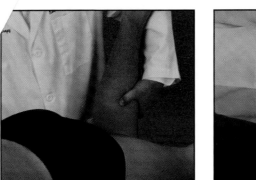

Medial head.   Lateral head.

MYOFASCIAL STRETCHES

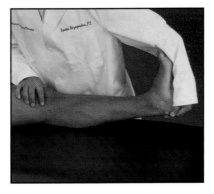

HOME EXERCISE PROGRAM

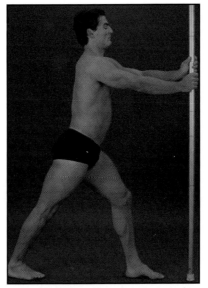

Notice that the knee of the stretched side is fully extended.

SOLEUS

ORIGIN

The head and a portion of the proximal body the fibula, and the medial border of tibia.

INSERTION

Through the Achilles' tendon to the calcaneus bone.

RPP

Achilles' tendon, calcaneus bone, belly of the muscle, sacroiliac joint.

TP

One HB above and three FB posterior to the medial malleolus.

MFS

The clinician facilitates dorsiflexion of the ankle with the knee bent.

PSS

Pain at the anterior ankle area.

HEP

The patient is in a standing position and stretches against a wall. He positions the foot to be stretched slightly behind the other foot and leans anteriorly, causing ankle dorsiflexion with the knee bent.

BIOMECHANICS OF INJURY

Climbing uphill, immobilization after ankle fractures.

CLINICAL NOTES

In cases of Achilles' tendonitis, the gastrocnemius should be treated together with the soleus and tibialis posterior muscles. Compression of the soleus canal may occur when patients use improper leg rests. This will result in numbness in the lower leg due to compression of the tibial artery, tibial vein, and posterior tibial nerve. The soleus can be myofascially involved and, thus, appropriate to be treated in cases of plantarfasciitis.

TRIGGER POINT THERAPY

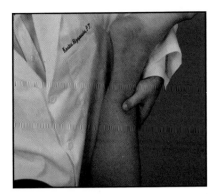

MYOFASCIAL STRETCHES

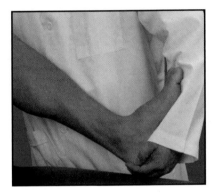

HOME EXERCISE PROGRAM

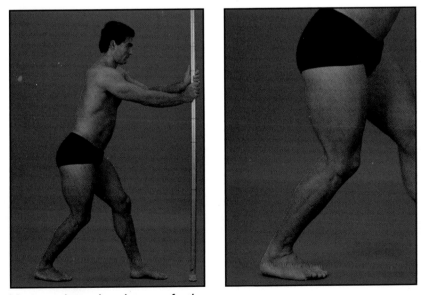

Notice that the knee of the stretched side is bent.

TIBIALIS ANTERIOR

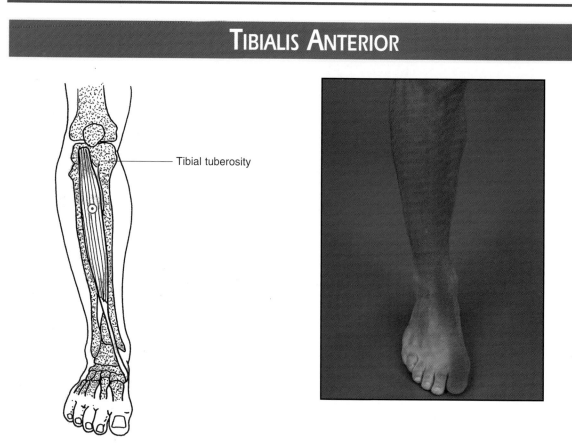

Tibial tuberosity

ORIGIN

Lateral condyle and superior half of the lateral surface of the tibia.

INSERTION

Base of the first metatarsal and cuneiform bones.

RPP

Anterior and medial aspects of the ankle and great toe.

TP

Four FB below the tibial tuberosity and one FB lateral to the tibial crest. Flat palpation.

MFS

Plantarflexion and eversion of the foot. The clinician facilitates foot movement.

PSS

Pain in the area of the lateral malleolus during foot eversion.

HEP

The patient is in a sitting position and facilitates stretch with the use of the hand.

BIOMECHANICS OF INJURY

Walking on uneven surfaces and uphill.

TRIGGER POINT THERAPY

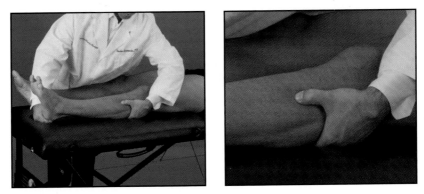

MYOFASCIAL STRETCHES

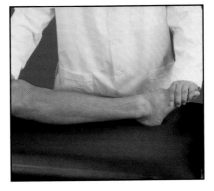

HOME EXERCISE PROGRAM

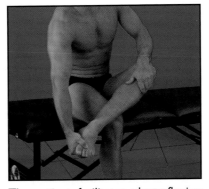

The patient facilitates plantarflexion and eversion.

TIBIALIS POSTERIOR

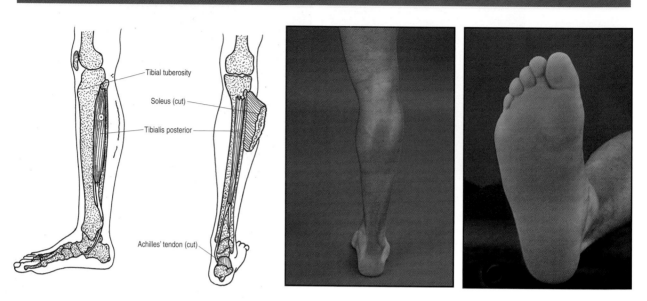

ORIGIN

Posterior surface of the tibia and superior two-thirds of the medial surface of the fibula.

INSERTION

Tuberosity of the navicular, cuboid, and cuneiforms.

RPP

Calf, Achilles' tendon, heel of the foot, along the belly of the muscle. On occasion, the muscle may cause shin splint pain.

TP

One HB below the tibial tuberosity and one FB medial to the medial edge of the tibia.

MFS

The clinician facilitates dorsiflexion and eversion of the ankle with the knee bent.

PSS

Pain at the anterior ankle area.

HEP

The patient is in a standing position and stretches against the wall. He positions the foot to be stretched slightly behind the other foot and leans anteriorly and laterally, causing ankle dorsiflexion and eversion with the knee bent.

BIOMECHANICS OF INJURY

Running or jogging on uneven ground. Hyperpronation of the feet will activate trigger points.

CLINICAL NOTES

In cases of Achilles' tendonitis, the gastrocnemius should be treated together with the soleus and tibialis posterior muscles. Causes shin splint pain in marathon runners. In cases of chronic heel spurs that have exacerbation of symptoms, treat the tibialis posterior. When tight and myofascially involved, the muscle will change the axis of rotation of the calcaneus, resulting in a new area of acute spur pressure.

TRIGGER POINT THERAPY

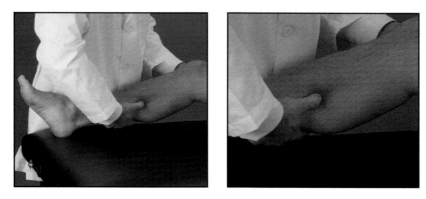

MYOFASCIAL STRETCHES

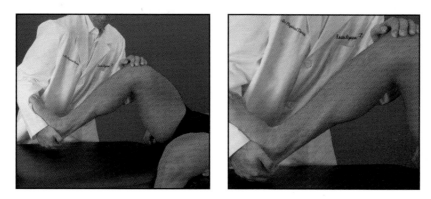

HOME EXERCISE PROGRAM

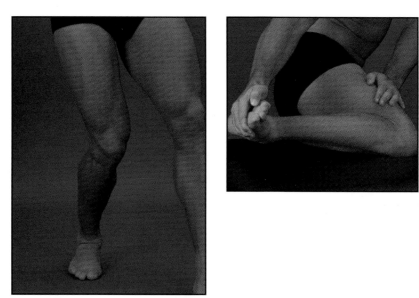

PERONEUS LONGUS

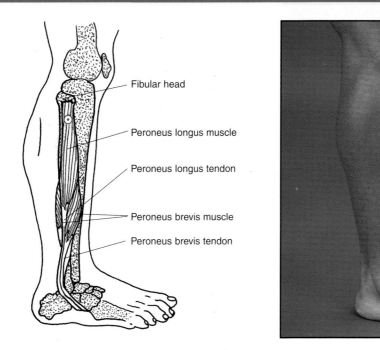

Fibular head

Peroneus longus muscle

Peroneus longus tendon

Peroneus brevis muscle

Peroneus brevis tendon

ORIGIN

Head and superior two-thirds of the lateral surface of the fibula.

INSERTION

Base of the first metatarsal bone and medial cuneiform bone.

RPP

Lateral aspect of the lower leg along the muscle belly.

TP

Three FB below the fibular head. Flat palpation.

MFS

Dorsiflexion with inversion of the foot. The clinician facilitates ankle movement.

PSS

Pain at the anterior and medial ankle areas.

HEP

Same as MFS. The patient facilitates stretch with the hand.

BIOMECHANICS OF INJURY

Prolonged immobilization after ankle fractures, wearing high heels, flat feet.

CLINICAL NOTES

The clinician should avoid contact with the neck of the fibular head, which is the passage for the common peroneal nerve.

TRIGGER POINT THERAPY

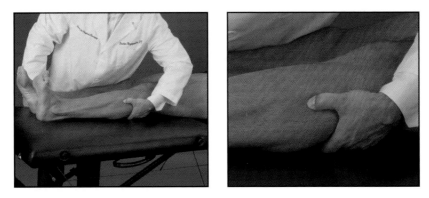

MYOFASCIAL STRETCHES

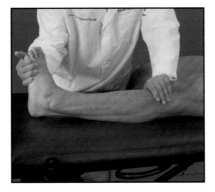

HOME EXERCISE PROGRAM

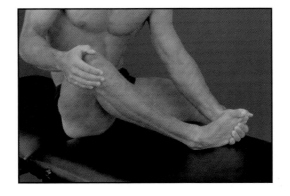

PERONEUS BREVIS

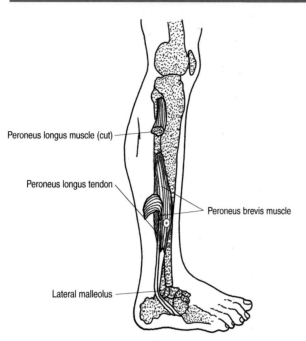

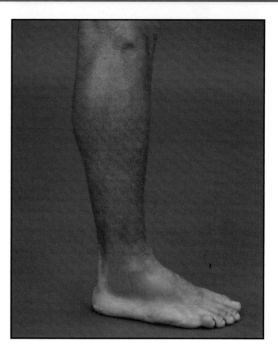

ORIGIN

Lower two-thirds of the fibula.

INSERTION

Base of the fifth metatarsal.

RPP

Lateral malleolus, lateral aspect of the foot.

TP

One HB proximal to the lateral malleolus and anterior to the peroneus longus tendon.

MFS

Dorsiflexion with inversion of the foot. The clinician facilitates ankle movement.

PSS

Pain at the anterior and medial ankle areas.

HEP

Same as MFS. The patient facilitates stretch with the hand.

BIOMECHANICS OF INJURY

Prolonged immobilization after ankle fractures, wearing high heels, flat feet.

CLINICAL NOTES

The trigger point is located under the tendon of the peroneus longus muscle. The clinician must move the thumb under the tendon to palpate the trigger point.

TRIGGER POINT THERAPY

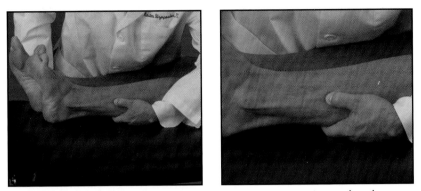

The clinician must locate the peroneus brevis trigger point under the peroneus longus tendon.

MYOFASCIAL STRETCHES

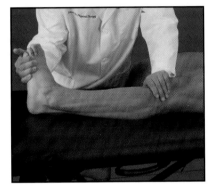

HOME EXERCISE PROGRAM

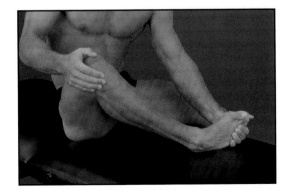

PERONEUS TERTIUS

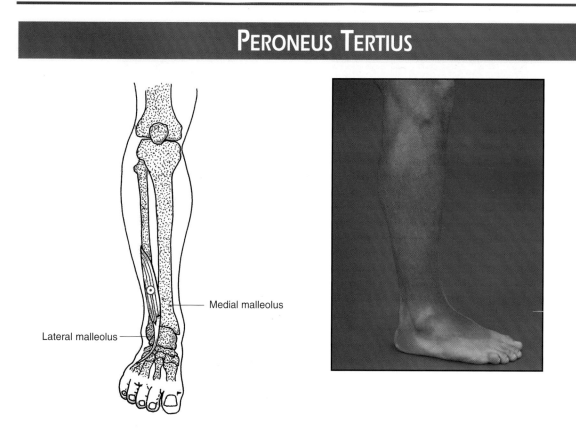

Lateral malleolus
Medial malleolus

ORIGIN

Lower one-third of the fibula.

INSERTION

Base of the fifth metatarsal head.

RPP

Anterior to the lateral malleolus and outer side of the heel.

TP

One HB above the bimalleolar line and two FB lateral to the tibia. Flat palpation.

MFS

The clinician facilitates plantarflexion of the ankle and inversion. Note: The peroneus tertius tendon passes anterior to the lateral malleolus.

PSS

Pain at the Achilles' tendon area.

HEP

Same as MFS. The patient facilitates stretch with the hand.

BIOMECHANICS OF INJURY

Same as other peronii.

TRIGGER POINT THERAPY

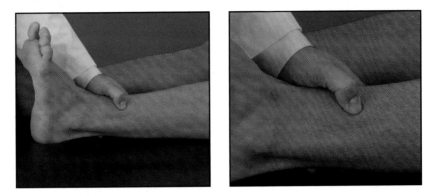

MYOFASCIAL STRETCHES

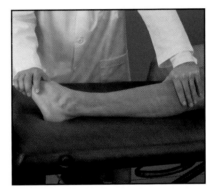

HOME EXERCISE PROGRAM

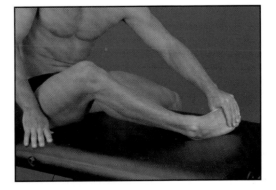

EXTENSOR DIGITORUM BREVIS

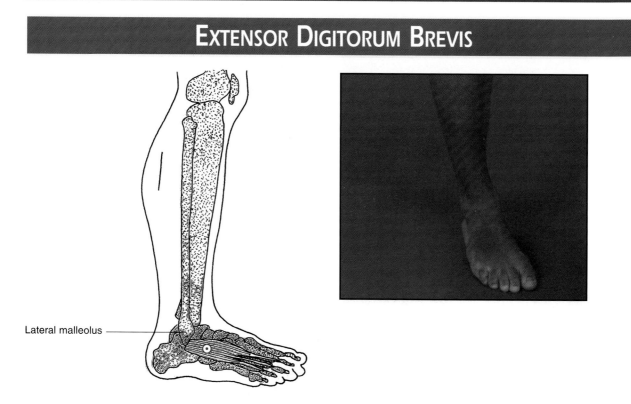

Lateral malleolus

ORIGIN

Upper and lateral surfaces of the calcaneus.

INSERTION

Tendon of the extensor digitorum longus of the second, third, and fourth toes.

RPP

Dorsum of the foot.

TP

Three FB distal to the lateral malleolus, parallel to the lateral border of the foot. Flat palpation.

MFS

Plantarflexion of the toes. The clinician facilitates stretch.

PSS

Not detected.

HEP

Same as MFS. The patient facilitates stretch with the hand.

BIOMECHANICS OF INJURY

Prolonged immobilization, tight shoes.

TRIGGER POINT THERAPY

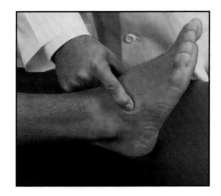

MYOFASCIAL STRETCHES

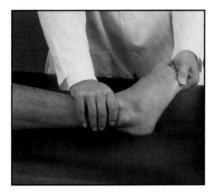

HOME EXERCISE PROGRAM

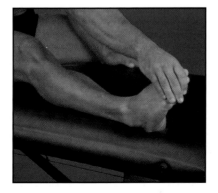

FLEXOR HALLUCIS BREVIS

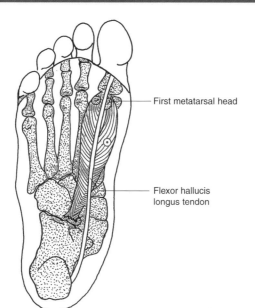

First metatarsal head

Flexor hallucis
longus tendon

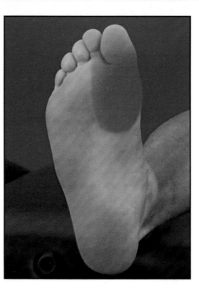

ORIGIN

Cuboid and cuneiform bones.

INSERTION

Base of the proximal phalanx of the great toe.

RPP

Region of both surfaces of the great toe.

TP

Two FB below the first metatarsal head.

MFS

Extension of the great toe. The clinician facilitates the stretch.

PSS

Not detected.

HEP

Same as MFS. The patient facilitates stretch with the hand.

BIOMECHANICS OF INJURY

Same as the abductor hallucis.

TRIGGER POINT THERAPY

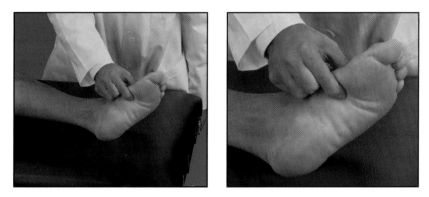

MYOFASCIAL STRETCHES

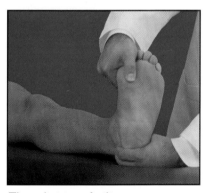

The clinician facilitates great toe extension while supporting above the first metatarsal head.

HOME EXERCISE PROGRAM

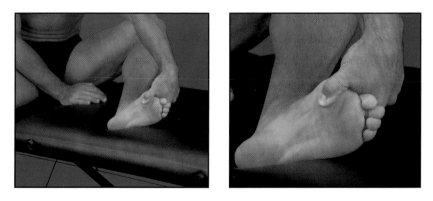

FLEXOR DIGITORUM BREVIS

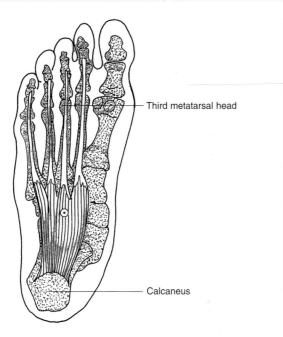

Third metatarsal head

Calcaneus

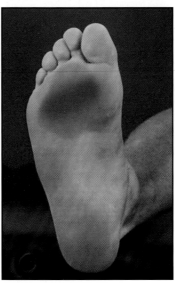

ORIGIN

Calcaneus and plantar aponeurosis.

INSERTION

Both sides of the middle phalanges of the lateral four toes.

RPP

Heads of the second to fourth metatarsals.

TP

Midway between the third metatarsal head and the calcaneus.

MFS

Extension of the four toes. The clinician facilitates stretching and stabilizes the calcaneus.

PSS

Not detected.

HEP

Same as MFS. The patient facilitates stretch with one hand while supporting the calcaneus with the other.

BIOMECHANICS OF INJURY

Same as the abductor hallucis.

TRIGGER POINT THERAPY

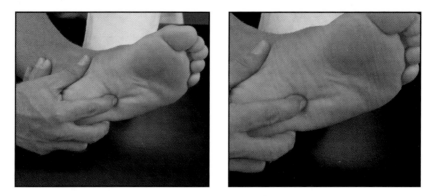

MYOFASCIAL STRETCHES

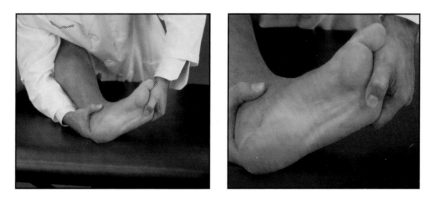

HOME EXERCISE PROGRAM

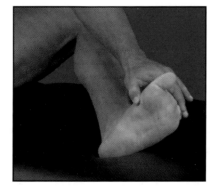

QUADRATUS PLANTAE

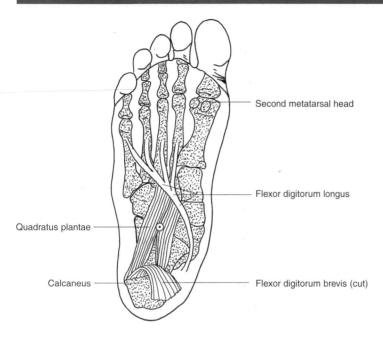

- Second metatarsal head
- Flexor digitorum longus
- Quadratus plantae
- Calcaneus
- Flexor digitorum brevis (cut)

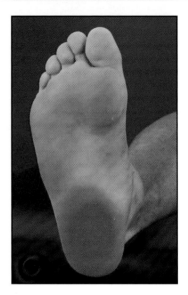

ORIGIN

Medial head—Medial surface of the calcaneus.
Lateral head—Lateral surface of the calcaneus.

INSERTION

Into the flexor digitorum longus tendon.

RPP

Plantar surface of the heel.

TP

Proximal and middle one-third of the line between the calcaneus and second metatarsal head.

MFS

Extension of the four toes. The clinician stabilizes the calcaneus bone with one hand and facilitates stretch with the other hand.

PSS

Not detected.

HEP

The patient applies the same stretch as MFS.

BIOMECHANICS OF INJURY

Restriction of toe movement, prolonged immobilization.

TRIGGER POINT THERAPY

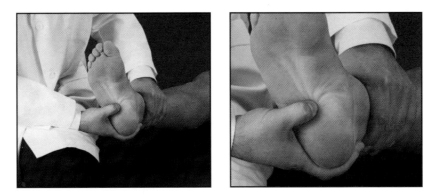

MYOFASCIAL STRETCHES

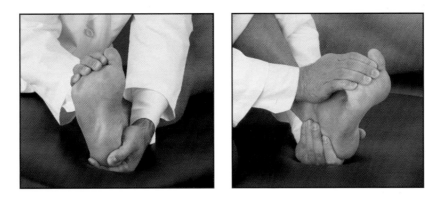

HOME EXERCISE PROGRAM

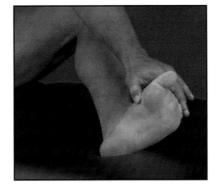

ADDUCTOR HALLUCIS

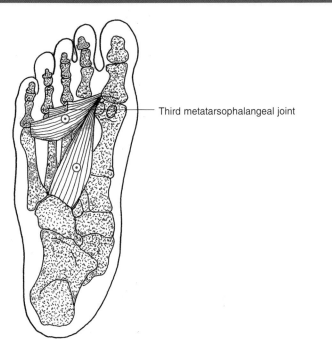

Third metatarsophalangeal joint

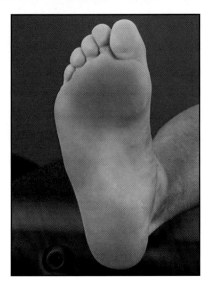

ORIGIN

Second to fourth metatarsals (oblique head) and third to fifth metatarsophalangeal joints (transverse head).

INSERTION

Proximal phalanx of the great toe.

RPP

Plantar surface of the forefoot.

TP

Over the belly of the muscle. Rarely a trigger point.

MFS

The clinician stabilizes the second to fifth metatarsals, and extends and abducts the great toe.

PSS

Not detected.

HEP

The patient applies the same stretch as MFS.

BIOMECHANICS OF INJURY

Restriction of toe movement, prolonged immobilization.

TRIGGER POINT THERAPY

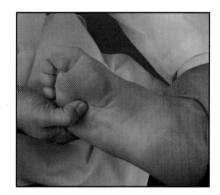

MYOFASCIAL STRETCHES

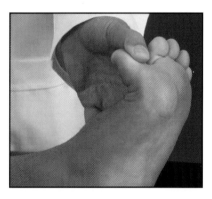

HOME EXERCISE PROGRAM

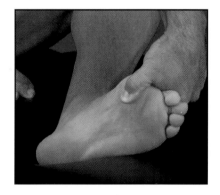

INDEX

EXPAND YOUR LIBRARY WITH THESE ESSENTIAL LEARNING TOOLS!

The Manual of Trigger Point and Myofascial Therapy offers a comprehensive therapeutic approach for the evaluation and treatment of myofascial pain and musculoskeletal dysfunction. With the most current information available and extensive full-color photographs and illustrations, this book is a necessity for the diagnosis and treatment of trigger point syndrome. To complement this exceptional text, SLACK Incorporated has just released two learning tools you will want to include in your library.

THE VIDEO OF TRIGGER POINT AND MYOFASCIAL THERAPY

VHS Videotape, 2001, ISBN 1-55642-557-0, Order #45570, $79.00

This two-hour long video presents a concise, comprehensive, and practical guide to the latest theories and interventions of myofascial trigger points. Watch and learn as the authors discuss theory and then present a detailed demonstration of their treatment techniques on a live model. Each of the main muscle systems in the body will be addressed, as the viewer will see an anatomical picture of the muscle in question in addition to the referred pain pattern. This is followed by an actual demonstration of the treatment techniques utilized, with verbal reinforcement pertaining to hand placements. Home exercises are also shown.

TRIGGER POINT AND MYOFASCIAL THERAPY POSTERS

2 Wall Charts, 24" x 36" each, 2001, ISBN 1-55642-556-2, Order #45562, $39.50

The Trigger Point and Myofascial Therapy Posters are two full-color posters that highlight most of the illustrations and photographs presented in the book, *The Manual of Trigger Point and Myofascial Therapy*. The photographs and illustrations included on these exceptional posters are not only of referred pain patterns but also reflect anatomy, trigger point techniques and myofascial stretches of key muscles throughout the body.

Title	Author	Book #	Price
The Video of Trigger Point and Myofascial Therapy	Kostopoulos, et al	45570	$79.00
Trigger Point and Myofascial Therapy Posters	Kostopoulos, et al	45562	$39.50

Subtotal $_____
NJ & CA Sales Tax* $_____
Handling Charge $4.50____
Total $_____

Name: _____ Email: _____

Address: _____

City: _____ State: _____ Zip: _____

Charge My: _____ American Express _____ Visa _____ Mastercard   Account #: _____

Expiration Date: _____ Signature: _____

Prices are subject to change. Shipping charges may apply. Shipping & handling charges are nonrefundable.

*Purchases in NJ and CA are subject to tax. Please add applicable state and local taxes.

CODE: 4A725

Mail Order Form To:
SLACK Incorporated
Professional Book Division
6900 Grove Road
Thorofare, NJ 08086-9864
Call: 800-257-8290 or 856-848-1000
Fax: 856-853-5991
Email: orders@slackinc.com
Visit Our World Wide Web: www.slackbooks.com